Praise for *the long hello*

"A sparse yet deeply affecting, poetic story of love and devotion . . . revealing moments of clarity, absurdity, wisdom, and connection that pierce and heal the heart."

—Lisa Genova

"Joy!"

—Maya Angelou

"Cathie Borrie is a great writer, and her exploration of life with Alzheimer's is deep, rich, nuanced, and soulful."

—Dr. Bill Thomas, author of *Second Wind*

"*The Long Hello* is a graceful dance between mother and daughter through the ever-changing rhythms of Alzheimer's disease. Beautiful and profound in its telling, this story reveals the depth of poetry and creativity that the changing brain can muster along its journey. One of my favorite books on the topic!"

—G. Allen Power, MD, author of *Dementia Beyond Drugs* and *Dementia Beyond Disease*

"Caregivers will recognize themselves both in the mix of light moments of connection and in the darker, unspeakable, intolerable emotions. . . . Borrie finds poetry in her mother's language, and teaches us all important lessons about the human experience of caring. . . . A beautifully written meditation on memory loss, suffering, hope, and love."

—Jed A. Levine, Executive Vice President and Director, Programs and Services, Alzheimer's Disease and Related Disorders, New York City, Inc.

"*The Long Hello* . . . offers a paradigm-shifting approach to maintaining relationship. Borrie enters deeply into her mother's world, and a poetic dialogue of mutual love and respect is the result. Should be required reading for everyone caring for people with dementia, and included in the syllabus of healthcare professionals learning how to do so."

—Marc Wortmann, Executive Director,
Alzheimer's Disease International

"Cathie Borrie has learned to respect the wisdom in her mother's free associations. *The Long Hello* will touch deeply all who love."
—Naomi Feil, author of *V/F Validation: The Feil Method* and *The Validation Breakthrough*, and Founder and Director in Chief, Validation Training Institute

"The warmth of her story combats the cold realities of ageism and negative stigma that have characterized the Alzheimer's and dementia world for too long. . . . I believe that Cathie's book should be made available to all caregivers, both lay and professional, as well as policy makers, researchers, and anyone else who advocates for this cause."

—Daniel C. Potts, MD, FAAN, Attending Neurologist,
Tuscaloosa VA Medical Center; Founder and
President, Cognitive Dynamics Foundation;
Medical Director, Dementia Dynamics, LLC

"The book's highly literary vision of disease is a powerful challenge to more detached clinical observations. . . . By approaching a parent's Alzheimer's in the spirit of hello rather than good-bye, Borrie is predisposed to pay attention—yet even then she's astonished at the words that emerge from her mother's mouth, almost as if aging could unlock the imagination and unleash a verbal force held back by logic and rationality."

—John Allemang, *Globe and Mail*

"Borrie captures the familiar cadence of repetition and the bizarre, yet touching conversations we share. We must live in their reality if we are to comfort them, and Cathie shows us how it can be done with love."

—Meryl Comer, President, Geoffrey Beene Foundation
Alzheimer's Initiative; Emmy-award winning reporter,
producer, moderator, talk show host; caregiver;
and Alzheimer's Association Board Member

"Cathie Borrie's groundbreaking lyrical memoir, *The Long Hello*, utilizes arrestingly poetic prose to create an ideological sea change in the way in which individuals and society at large view the experience of Alzheimer's, shinning new light on the rich emotional and intellectual ways of being that are newly possible in the altering world of the dementia mind."

—Francesca Rosenberg, Director, Community and Access Programs, Museum of Modern Art

"A moving and amazing breakthrough of a book."

—Lynn Jackson, co-founder of the Dementia Advocacy and Support Network International (DASNI)

"Ebullient, feisty, vulnerable, and dumbstruck by the circumstances of her life, Cathie Borrie uses the magical lens of her mother's Alzheimer's disease to examine her role of dutiful daughter. With her theatrical sense of timing . . . and her skill as a poet, Borrie writes a page-turning memoir of a whole family. . . . I read this book right straight through, with all the other things I had to do, standing at attention for *The Long Hello*. . . . Miraculously, Borrie both replicates her mother's thinking and used it as a threshold into her own remembering."

—Molly Peacock, author of *Paradise, Piece by Piece*, and *The Paper Garden: Mrs. Delany Begins Her Life's Work at 72*

"A masterpiece . . . An absorbing and fascinating account, beautifully written and of value to all engaged in the care of Alzheimer's patients—from caregiving relatives to those providing medical and social services to the ever-growing number of patients."

—Dr. D. A. Henderson, Professor of Medicine and Public Health, University of Pittsburgh; and University Distinguished Service Professor and Dean Emeritus, The Johns Hopkins Bloomberg School of Public Health

"What Cathie Borrie did for her mother was wonderful. . . . What she has done for readers is inspiring. The actions are matched by the luminous prose. This book is memoir at its best."

—*Vancouver Sun*

"*The Long Hello* is an amazing neo-existentialist vision, profoundly layered with love, death, agony, exquisite language, loneliness, and more love. I was overwhelmed by the filmic, sensuous imagery, the emotional force of such a raw interweaving of past and present. From somewhere (out) here, Cathie Borrie has created a book of shimmering truth, a narrative of a life lived where we are, and a life lived on 'the other side of here.'"

—Christian Xatrec, artist, Director of the
Emily Harvey Foundation, NYC

"Toward the end, as her mother copes with a brutal cough, Borrie gently touches her chest: 'Is there enough compassion in there?' her mother asks. 'Yes, Mum,' Borrie answers. 'It's full, beautiful.' The same can be said for her daughter's remarkable book."

—Anne Kingston, *Maclean's*

"Filled with insights that will be of interest to caregivers and their families. Lyrical and evocative, it is about remembering and forgetting, presence and absence, holding on and letting go. . . . Cathie Borrie is a gifted storyteller, and she has written a memorable book about love and loss."

—Jeffery Berman, author and Distinguished Teaching
Professor of English at the State University of New York

"Cathie Borrie's heartwarming message will have you finding joy as a caregiver—even in your darkest, most difficult times. . . . I am very impressed with her ability to touch and inspire others."

—Steve Harrison, *Radio-TV Interview Report*,
Million Dollar Author Club

the long hello

the long hello

Memory, My Mother, and Me

CATHIE BORRIE

Arcade Publishing • New York

First US Edition 2016

Arcade Publishing books may be purchased in bulk at special discounts for
sales promotion, corporate gifts, fund-raising, or educational purposes. Special
editions can also be created to specifications. For details, contact the Special
Sales Department, Arcade Publishing, 307 West 36th Street, 11th Floor, New
York, NY 10018 or arcade@skyhorsepublishing.com.

Arcade Publishing® is a registered trademark of Skyhorse Publishing, Inc.®,
a Delaware corporation.

Visit our website at www.arcadepub.com.
Visit the author's site at www.cathieborrie.com.

10 9 8 7 6 5 4 3 2 1

Library of Congress Cataloging-in-Publication Data

Names: Borrie, Cathie, author.
Title: The long hello: memory, my mother, and me / Cathie Borrie.
Description: First U.S. edition. | New York: Arcade Publishing, [2015] |
Previously published: Vancouver: Nightwing Press, c2010.
Identifiers: LCCN 2015043983|
ISBN 9781628726640 (hardback) | ISBN 9781628726671 (ebook)
Subjects: LCSH: Borrie, Cathie. | Borrie, Joan—Mental health. | Alzheimer's
disease—Patients—Care—British Columbia—Vancouver. | Alzheimer's
disease—Patients—Family relationships—British Columbia—Vancouver. |
Mothers and daughters—British Columbia—Vancouver—Biography. |
Vancouver (B.C.)—Biography. | BISAC: BIOGRAPHY & AUTOBIOGRAPHY /
Personal Memoirs. | SOCIAL SCIENCE / Disease & Health Issues.
Classification: LCC RC523.2 .B67 2016 | DDC 362.1968/310092—dc23
LC record available at http://lccn.loc.gov/2015043983

Jacket design by Laura Klynstra
Cover illustration: iStock

Printed in the United States of America

the long hello

Forty years after his death, I dream my brother and I are walking arm in arm down a country lane in the late afternoon sun. He's close to twenty in my dream and heavier, taller. I can't stop crying.

"Hughie, I've missed you so much. I just love you so much."

He looks down, squeezes me tight.

"I know, Cath. I know."

Every day I sit with my mother and watch the sea. There's a row of birds perched on an errant log—cormorant, cormorant, seagull, heron. Crow.

"Cathie, sometimes I drift off for ten minutes and I don't know where I've gone."

"Does that bother you, Mum?"

"No, it doesn't. Are you my daughter?"

We watch frantic wing-flitting at her bird feeder. Chickadees, starlings, sparrows. A house finch, brown-striped.

"Cath, I think it's a finch, it's only . . . oh—a finch a finch a finch! Are they trying to tell you they aren't in there? What are they trying to say?"

"To say . . . ? I don't know."

"I think there's something, they're trying to get something across, aren't they, love?"

Bird-pecking at the feeder. I tap on the window.
"Chick-a-dee-dee-dee, chick-a-dee-dee-dee. How do you think birds get their names?"

"I don't know."

"What shall I call myself? What name?"

"Don't you know?"

"Yes, but I'd like a different name."

"Well, I like Hugh or Cath but I think Hugh is better. More suitable."

"But you won't ever forget me, will you?"

"As if I ever could."

Starlings replace chickadees. The seed is getting low.

"What do you think is the most important thing, Mum? I mean, a good thing?"

"Understanding."

"And what about the rest of your life? What's your thinking on the rest of your life?"

"Oh gosh, there can't be much left of it can there, Cath? What will I be, sixty-six?"

"You're going to be eighty-six."

"Oh yeah, eighty-six."

"How old am I?"

"Oh about sixty, sixty and the pen you're holding. I'm sixty-two or -three, the age I quickly got to."

"How would you like to live out the remainder of your days?"

"I don't know, it fills me with horror. The same as what I'm doing over there only I'll be better. I'll be flying down the hill in my jacket!"

We listen to Bach.

"Did someone take the place of A-flat minor? You know, I think about the radio, listen to the radio, and I wonder if Cath is listening, too."

"You mean . . . you wonder about me when you're listening to the radio?"

"Yes. It's the only time."

Prelude no. 1 in C Major. My mother sighs, closes her eyes.

"What was he thinking? What was Bach thinking?"

"What's the nicest thing about you?"

"Nothing."

"Okay, what's the second-nicest thing about you?"

"My love of music, my love of good music. In fact it might be the first thing. Do you know what I had last night?"

"What?"

"Two lots of the London Conservatory taken away."

"What do you like least about yourself?"

"All the things I could do and wanted to do and didn't do because I couldn't be bothered."

"You always loved music, didn't you?"

"It was Mother who made me compete. Once, when I was six, at that big hotel downtown, a man lifted me up onto the piano stool and I was so mad because I could have got up by myself. Mother never forgave me for quitting, but I was just so nervous. I hated it. After I left, my piano teacher told Mother that the German adjudicator asked her where the little golden-haired girl was, the one with music in her ears."

Our eyes scan the sea.

"There's a huge freighter coming in. I wonder where it's from."

My mother squints.

"It's coming in too full, you can't see the Plimsoll line."

"You have a good eye."

"Yes, but is it the right eye?"

"You're feeling better today, aren't you?"

"Yes."

"Because?"

"Because it's all coming in and none going out."

Four cruise ships leave the harbor for Alaska one after the other.

"Here they come, *Norwegian Wind, Veendam, Dawn Princess, Radiance of the Seas.* They're getting bigger every year."

"I've been on one of those ships and spent a whole morning up on the bridge. You should see the instruments. Wow!"

"Which do you like better, the sea or the sky?"

"The sea."

"Because?"

"You can swim in it."

"And?"

"It's always out there for you. It's always there."

I feel guilty if I don't visit her every day, all day, guilty every moment I'm not with my mother. Worrying all the time that she'll fall and not be able to call me, not remember the personal alarm pendant around her neck. Worry she'll be lonely. Most of her friends are dead, and visits from family dwindling. For a long time she won't let me hire anyone to help.

"I like my own company, I always have. So did Dad, it's one of the reasons we got on so well. I think the nicest thing about it is that I like people and they come to see me and they want to come and see you. Everything is on my head, you know. I don't want them to come and see me, or you. I'm a loner, darling, but those fancy things, they like it. It's just that I like it best when you're here, love."

"But Mum, I can't keep—"

"We don't need anyone else, lovey. I like it the way it is."

When she can no longer walk, I have to hire live-in caregivers, then worry, knowing how much she hates strangers in her home. Worry about what they're doing, not doing, and spend as much time with her as before we had help. I fire one when I learn she isn't talking to my mother. Another I'm never quite sure about quits while my mother is dying. The best, a quiet gentle soul. The one who stays.

Mum wakes up my brother and me in the middle of the night because we have to move to the country to live with her parents. We're to put a few of our favorite things into a plastic bag. My brother is eight and wants to bring his bike, but there isn't room. I'm five and bring my favorite doll but she wets herself so I have to remember all her diapers.

"Hurry, Hughie. Come on, Cath. Uncle Hugh's waiting."

"What's the matter, Mum? Where are we going? It's so dark."

I'm scared.

She rushes back and forth from the house to the car carrying paper bags and suitcases that she hands her brother to put in the trunk. No time to pack our books, Mum's records and sheet music, photo albums.

"I feel awful bringing you out this late, Hugh, and you'll miss work tomorrow."

"It's all right, Jo."

"It's just that he's . . . he's drunk most of the time now and I was afraid he might do something, I mean, to the children."

"I wish I'd known. I want you all to be safe, that's all that matters, kid."

"You're the only one I'd call, Hugh."

We hurry out to my uncle's car running in the driveway. I climb into the backseat next to my brother. He's wearing his cowboy hat and staring out the window and I want to hold his hand but he wouldn't like that. I look back at our house as we drive away to see if our dad is watching or running after us. It's pitch-black. It feels funny leaving him behind.

"Where's Daddy?"

"He's not home right now, darling. You have to be a big girl for Mum, all right?"

"But he won't know where we are. How will he find us? We should go back for Daddy. Let's go home now, Mum. Mum?"

"Cathie, stop! Be quiet!"

My mum has never shouted at me like that. I don't know what to do. We drive to my grandparents' in the dark. No one speaks.

A few months after we move in with our grand-parents our father comes to visit my brother and me. When I see his car come around the corner I run out and wrap myself around him.

"Daddy! Daddy!"

He pats the top of my head. My brother stands beside my mother, watching. We drive into town to get ice-cream cones and Mum comes too, but she sits in the back. My gran says our dad isn't allowed to take my brother and me anywhere alone.

"Why not, Gran?"

"Because he drinks and he can't be trusted. Do you know he's never sent your mother a dime?"

Our father's allowed to visit my brother and me twice a month. He never comes again.

For lunch I make fruit salad and cottage cheese and one piece of whole-wheat toast. I stand at my mother's kitchen window cutting up fruit and look out at the day. It's raining. A raven watches me from his perch on the power line as the wind whisks wave tips into frothy white manes. I try not to think about where I am and what I do all day or the things I used to do and miss most—working, studying, canoeing, movies. Men.

She has her lunch on a TV table in the den.

"How are you, Mum?"

"I'm sort of dragging myself through."

"What are you dragging yourself through?"

"Oh, wheat fields and sticky things. Someone's pinning me all together. Oh yes, yes, I'm very, very clear. When that girl Cathie phoned this morning I thought, what's she phoning me for?"

"Cathie? But I'm Cathie—"

"Then I heard her say, 'Oh, because it's a day.' But she didn't say the right name. Anyway, he went into sing and you went into sing, didn't you?"

"Into . . . sing? Um, I guess I did. Mum, I miss you."

"You know, I just stamp my foot and there she isn't."

"She? Oh. You know, even though I see you every day I still miss you."

"Then my daughter Cathie came back to this side when she was through over there. I guess she was through and I was so surprised and thrilled and we had tea together and it was nifty."

"Your daughter? Well, how would you like us to be related?"

"I think we're doing fine in the water."

I tell people I'm still working and making money but I'm not. Try to ignore the tightness in my chest from having to move so slowly when I like moving fast, and the creeping sense of captivity that sits heavy in my gut.

My mother sits on her couch with her eyes closed.

"Would you like to have a little rest?"

"Okay, dear. But where are you going to sit? And then you're going to go away with Dad, aren't you, and I'll be all alone."

"I never go away with Dad."

"Oh, that's good."

"You seem so tired . . . are you giving up?"

"No, I don't give up. I don't know how to do it."

"Neither do I."

I draw the curtains.

"How was your day?"

"It's very hard for me to tell you because when you say, How have you been today, Mum? I try to think, and I can't think of anything. I don't know what I did this morning, I have no idea."

"Oh. Maybe a better question would be—how are you right now?"

"Well, I'm fine, just fine. Yes, it's a good, a better question to come for me."

"You look like a little porcelain doll lying there."

"Does it, does it look just like china?"

"Yes, just perfect."

"Well, that's good. Somebody's got to be perfect."

When we move in with Gran and Grampy my mum has to go back to work. She used to teach piano lessons to kids on our street because our father didn't make enough money, but now she has to go work in an office. Nobody else's mother works and I wish my mum could stay home, too. She says no one likes her boss.

"He gets mad all the time and someone's always in tears. One of the girls thinks he drinks."

Grampy wants her to find another job.

"There aren't any other jobs right now, Dad. But oh dear, the office is in a mess. The old files take up too much space, memos go unanswered, and the equipment is always breaking down, but he won't spend the money to repair it or have it replaced."

One day he shouts at her for being late with a letter and she tells us all about it at dinner.

"He just stood at the door of his office shouting—everyone could hear. But I know he never dictated that letter to me, so I marched right into his office and let him have it. I said, I quit! You don't like me,

I know you don't. I can't do anything right, there's no point in me staying here any longer."

My grandmother is horrified.

"Oh, Jo, you didn't."

"Then what, Mum, then what?"

"Well, I couldn't believe it, I was so embarrassed . . . but I started to cry."

Mum never cries in front of anyone.

"I tried to stop but I couldn't. I thought he was going to fire me, but instead he handed me one of his hankies and told me he couldn't stand to see a woman cry. I told him I was the only one in the office who defended him and that everyone hated working there. He said if I stayed I could take over the office and do anything I wanted. He'd give me a raise so I could send little Hughie to boarding school and order new equipment. Anything, if only I stay."

My mum stays. Her boss gives her a really big raise and even a key to the vault. She buys us all presents and picks out a pair of earrings for herself—two dangly half-moons in silver, gold, and black.

"Two dollars! I feel so guilty."

She sends me to private school as a daygirl and my brother, with the help of a bursary, to a boarding school only an hour away. My brother hasn't been doing well in school and my mother thinks he'll do better around other boys and male teachers. She says he's too old to be around just us and that my grandparents don't have the energy for an eleven-year-old boy.

Every Sunday we drive to his new school and bring him home for the day. One afternoon he cuts his hand on a shell at the beach and when I see his blood in the bathroom sink I can't stop crying.

"Oh, Mum. My Hughie . . ."

"He's already back outside with his friends! Shall we surprise him with his favorite chocolate cake for dessert, darling?"

During the drive back Hughie and I see who can count the most cows or sheep and sometimes we try to guess when a mile has gone by. Mostly my brother wins. When we drop him off I look out the back window and wave and wave until I can't see him anymore.

My mum works really hard to save enough money to buy me a bike and all summer long my friends and I ride past farms with horses and cows grazing in the fields. We all like horses the best and when we make clicking sounds and kissing noises they trot over and butt our legs with their heads trying to get at the bits of carrots and apples hidden deep within our pockets. They graze on our flat outstretched hands, their big rubbery lips tickling. I wipe their slimy spit on my shorts and for the rest of the day cup my hands over my face. Breathe in horse.

When we aren't out biking we play horses and run through the woods jumping over logs we've set up across narrow twisty trails. I always rear up, snorting and pawing at the dirt. I'm lead horse, tall and fast and wild. Unbreakable.

My mother and I lie side by side on her bed and look out at the day. Cradled between steel side rails we have a view of the maple tree and the crow-peppered holly bushes.

"The trees outside your window are so lush, Mum."

"Yes, lush, and the fish jumping out of the sea. You are like the sea. Tide going in, tide going out, storms, beautiful sky . . . full of fish."

She strokes my hair.

"All I ever wanted was to be a mother. Everywhere I went people would stop to tell me what beautiful babies you were—both of you with curly brown hair and big blue eyes—my little darlings. You always wanted to be where your brother was and if you couldn't find him you'd go round and knock on all the neighbors' doors until you did. Dorothy would call to say you were over there so I wouldn't worry. You just marched right in and asked if your boy was there."

"Really? Didn't he mind?"

"Oh no, love. He was always looking out for you. I was so excited when you were born. I wanted a little girl so badly, my very own little doll that I could dress up in pretty things. I called you Catherine but I should have called you Sporty!"

Bird-scrambling at the feeder.

"Have they enough seed?"

"Yes, there's still plenty, Mum."

"Your father came to the hospital after you were born. You were a cesarean and your sweet little face didn't have a mark on it! He was drunk, and threw a book at my stomach."

I cover my ears.

"Please don't tell me this story again, Mum. You have to stop telling me this story."

Five minutes later, she's forgotten. Begins again.

"Your father drank. He was jealous of you and little Hughie and said he wished you'd never been born. How could a father say that? His parents drank, both of them, and his brother. They'd all come for dinner, drunk when they arrived. It was awful. They sent your father to boarding school when he was only six, just a baby, really. You don't do that to a child, do you, Cath?"

A raven tries to land on the feeder but it's too heavy, flies away.

"One day your brother was asleep in his crib and your father came up from the basement. I made him coffee. He went down the hall to Hughie's room and ran the silver christening cup back and forth across the crib rails. Hughie woke up, screaming. Your father yelled at me, 'Can't you shut that stupid baby up? Shut that baby up!'"

"Mum—"

"I didn't know what to do. We didn't talk about things in those days. I should have known what to do. I thought it would pass, that he'd come around."

"Oh look, the chickadees are back—look."

"You used to wait at the window for him, 'Daddy! Daddy!' He'd push you away when you tried to get on his lap. The look on your little face . . . I tried to get you to stop, but you wouldn't. The lawyer said no one would believe me because he was so good at hiding his drinking and fooled everybody, even AA, and that I'd lose half my friends. Don't cry, darling, don't cry. Oh deary me, I did the best I could with the brains I had in my head."

She sips her tea.

"Is all this real or pretend?"

"I don't know. What would you like it to be?"

"Pretend."

"All right. It's Wednesday, so that means . . . yes, it's pretend."

"Oh good. But it's kind of a lousy time, isn't it?"

As soon as I'm home I call to say good night.

"Hi Mum, it's Cath. What are you doing?"

"I'm waiting for you. . . . I'm just here waiting for you."

"But I just got home. I was just over there."

"Over here?"

"Yes . . . never mind. I'll call first thing in the morning, okay?"

"Where are you? I couldn't find you."

"I'm home, I'm at my home. I'm fine."

"I thought I'd left you in the living room, all alone."

I drink two glasses of my favorite red wine, eat two bars of dark chocolate, swallow one and a half sleeping pills, and sink down into nothing. I crawl into bed in my clothes, pull the radio up beside me, and tune in my favorite all-night talk show. Tonight's program features government conspiracies, CIA subterfuge, contrail theory, alien abductions. The window is wide open, my bedroom is freezing. I wrap the sheet around my face, a shroud. As far as my mind can see there is nothing.

Everywhere.

My new favorite thing.

In the summer Mum takes my brother and me swimming down at the bay. We dive through each other's legs and sometimes he closes his legs just as I'm going through, pinning me tight. When I come up for air I'm really mad at him and splash water in his face as hard as I can and then we laugh. I carry Mum around in the shallow salty water and my brother swims after us, tickling her feet.

"Oh, Hughie, stop it! You know I can't stand any-one touching my feet! Hughie!"

My brother and I carve out beds deep in the sand. Trace imaginary letters on each other's backs.

"An F!"

"Was that a J?"

I always get the M and W mixed up.

After dinner my gran and I often go for long walks along the country road. She knows the names of all the plants we see along the way and spots flowers no one else can see.

"Look at that little darling tucked away under the branch. Did you know that lady's slipper is really a tiny fairy shoe? The fairies dance all night long and when the sun comes up they hang their shoes back up to dry."

She shows me where they danced the night before, pointing with her walking stick at the flattened circular markings in the grass.

"Look, darling, do you see the fairy ring?"

I don't but badly want to. "Where, Gran? Where?"

"There, see that piece of grass? It's all stomped down with their dancing. Naughty fairies, up all night."

On hot summer afternoons I lay my dolls down on a blanket in the backyard and play house. My gran helps me fill a large plastic bowl with warm water to use as a bathtub for my babies.

"Dry very carefully between their little toes and behind their ears and dress them as quickly as you can. You don't want them to catch cold, do you, darling?"

After their bath my dolls and I lie down together under an umbrella and take a pretend nap. My gran tucks us in.

"What a good little mother you are."

The spring my mother has a good spell I spend time with an artist, a wood-turner. While he works I paddle my canoe in search of treasures and find a discarded bird's nest. At night we curl up on the couch listening to Coltrane and Metheny.

When my mother gets worse I stop visiting my wood-turner.

Before I leave, he makes me a half-moon treasure box turned from a cedar burl, and during long winter nights with my mother, I breathe in the earthy scent of wood and oil, dreaming of trees and stones and bark and the buttery slice of my paddle slipping into the sea.

When my mother can't get in and out of the bath anymore I wear a green garbage bag over my clothes and help her in the shower. We're both embarrassed.

"I don't mind, Mum. You gave me lots of baths when I was a baby."

"I'm not a baby."

"I didn't mean . . ."

I can't get the room warm enough, the water temperature right. She shivers, her thin, dry skin flaking off on the towel. I feel sick.

"Love, do be careful. Don't let me fall!"

"I'm sorry, I'm sorry."

When we can't manage showers anymore she goes to the Seniors' Day Centre for her weekly bath and hair wash in a bright, heated room. There's a towel warmer, lavender-scented suds, kind staff, a yellow rubber duck.

Once a month we visit her doctor for advice, prescriptions, and for the kind words she makes sure my mother hears during every visit.

"You're doing so well."

"I know, I'm much better."

"Yes, you are. I just want to listen to your chest today."

"Oh yeah, you and all the other boys."

"Good one! I know you had some trouble with that pill I gave you and I'd like to try another one."

"I just can't remember things. My mind, it's all mixed up."

"Mrs. B., Parkinson's does that in some people, so I'm hoping this drug will help with that. I'm really very impressed with how you're doing."

My mother beams and for the rest of the day she goes over and over what the doctor has told her.

"Did you hear what she said? She thinks I'm doing really well and I am, you know. I'm better every day."

"She's really pleased with you."

"Do you really think so? Oh my."

When she no longer remembers the visits I tell her what the doctor has said.

"She said she was really pleased with you and that you are doing a really good job."

"And then what did I say?"

"You told her that you were trying very hard."

"I did? Well, that sounds silly."

"Um, oh, and then you thanked her for her kindness and for being such a good doctor."

"Oh, that's better. Yes, I like that better."

When we get home I put on the kettle.

"Are you happy?"

"Yes."

"How happy?"

"I'm very happy."

"Because?"

"Because I have no faith in anyone."

I start to close the blinds.

"Leave the curtains open so I can see the birds."

"How does one look after a bird?"

"Unless it's very tame, you can't. You know, I'm twice bitten and three times shy and I can't remember. Listen—a bird!"

"What are the birds saying?"

"They're chirping."

"In a language?"

"In their language. In an upside-down language."

Wedged tightly between the kitchen cupboard and the warm flank of the woodstove I watch my gran bake bread. When she stops to rest I wrap my arms around her waist and breathe in her flour-dusted, food-fragranced apron. She squeezes me tight, kisses the top of my head.

"Gran's little darling, aren't you?"

On summer afternoons I sit in the sun and watch my grandfather in his garden, mowing, digging, planting. Watch him mix lye soap and tobacco in a pot of boiling water.

"Grampy, why do you put tobacco in there?"

"Insects don't like the taste of tobacco. This will keep them away from my plants."

"But it won't hurt them, will it?"

"Oh no. Would you like Grampy to set aside a small patch of earth, pet, so you can have a little garden all your own?"

My grandfather, old and thin, works in his garden all day long, a home-rolled cigarette dangling from his mouth. My grandmother shouts at him from the kitchen window.

"Don't put that camellia under the tree, it won't get enough sun!"

My grandfather keeps digging, doesn't look up. Plants the camellia under the tree.

When he gets sick my mum learns how to give him shots for pain until he has to move to the nursing home and then she visits him every day after work and on the weekends. I'm allowed to visit him Sunday afternoons. He lies in a narrow bed with a white sheet tucked high up under his chin. On warm days he sits outside on the veranda in a wheelchair. He doesn't talk very much and sometimes catches his breath then squeezes his eyes tight shut.

"Grampy, you should have seen the hornets' nest under the eave!"

"Mind you don't get stung now, darling."

"It's all right, Grampy, somebody got rid of it, but I was so mad because Gran made me stay in the house the whole time."

On the day he dies, Mum picks me up from school.

"I have sad news, Cath."

I crawl into the backseat.

"Grampy died today. It's good, lovey, no more suffering for Grampy."

After my grampy dies I climb the tree that shades my grandparents' garage and wait for my mum to come home from work every day. From my favorite branch I can see the water tower across the road and the low-lying farms scattered throughout the valley. I lean against the rough, pine-scented bark, my fingers sticky with pitch.

After Grampy dies my brother moves into his room and I'm allowed to move into Hughie's, but I want to be in the same room as my mum. I'm allowed to read for half an hour before I have to go to sleep, and beside my bed there's a small wooden shelf where I keep my china horse and Dalmatian dog and all my favorite books: *Daddy-Long-Legs*, *The Incredible Journey*, *The Secret Garden*, *Anne of Green Gables*, *Black Beauty*.

I listen to kitchen sounds in the dark—to murmured conversations I can't quite hear, to broom-swooshing, the dull thud of closing cupboards, and the sharp clean clink of china. My mum leaves the bedroom curtains open so I can see the stars against the black night. I can't sleep with all the grasshopper and cricket chirping.

The spring my brother turns thirteen he won't let me in his room anymore.

"Get out! I don't want you in here. Get out!"

"But Hughie, I just want to say hi and things."

"Get out!"

My brother has never yelled at me like this. My mother tries to talk to him.

"Come on, Hughie, she just wants to visit. She won't stay long."

"Get out of my room! Just fuck off."

Mum and I go back to her bedroom and sit on the bed. She starts crying.

"Oh Cath . . ."

"Hughie didn't mean it. All the boys at school say it, they hate girls. It's okay, Mum, they say that to everyone."

One weekend Mum goes back to the city to visit friends and Gran makes her a pink wool dress with a matching jacket.

"Oh, Jo, you're so thin."

At dinner she sits beside a man, a widower, who will become our second father. He's twenty-two years older than she is, but Mum says he's in very good shape. He's already raised a family and his daughter and son are just a little younger than my mother. His grandchildren are the same ages as my brother and me.

"He used to come to meetings at the office where I worked, more than twenty years ago! He was always so nice to everyone and it didn't matter if you were the head of a big company or the doorman, he was always the same—nice to everyone. We all thought he was marvelous."

After the dinner party he starts calling my mother every Sunday and sends postcards from the cities he visits on his business trips.

"He's very successful and all sorts of women have been after him but he says he likes my spunk. Things

37

are going to be much better now, my darlings—you'll see."

He stays in a motel when he comes to visit and always brings us presents. He gives me a jewelry box with a gold satin lining that plays Brahms's Lullaby while a ballerina in a pink tutu twirls around and around.
"Look at my card, Mum! He wrote, 'With love.'"

He buys Hughie a shiny black-and-red guitar and my brother practices in his room for hours and hours, and during the next visit he puts on a show and plays the same song three times in a row.
Hughie and I don't spend any time with him alone because his visits are too short but we like the idea of having a new important father. Everyone we know has a father and we like getting all the presents.

I'm trying to get my mother to the bathroom. Trying to maneuver her wheelchair around the tight corners. I've sent the caregiver out for a break and told her she doesn't need to be back until dinner. I send her out for long breaks most days.

"Hurry, I'm not going to make it."

I start to lift her onto the toilet seat but my left hip lets me down. I can't manage her light weight, can't make the turn, and knock her leg against the bathroom cabinet. Drops of blood drip onto the beige mat but I can't let her go to get a bandage. My shirt is stuck to my back.

"I'm sorry. I'm sorry. I can't do a goddamn thing right. I'm such a stupid goddamn idiot!"

"Oh, love, your language."

"I'm sorry, I'm sorry."

"Are you crying? You're a darling to look after me so well. A sweet, sweet, darling."

"I'm not, Mum. I . . ."

"Yes you are, yes you are. My great big love. You pass on so many compliments I hate to let you go."

June. A clear hot day noisy with shrieks, barking, and the cracking pop of a starting gun. My right leg is tied to my mum's left leg with strips of old fabric, our arms wrapped tightly around each other's waists. We scuttle over to the edge of the lime-white starting line.

"Take your marks—get set—go!"

We've signed up for the three-legged race, signed up for all the races. During morning assembly our headmistress lectures us on the meaning of Sports Day.

"Now just remember, girls, today is all about doing your very best, being good sports, and having fun."

We want to win.

We've been practicing for weeks in my grandparents' backyard. My mother outlines our race strategy.

"Now remember, the first step is the most important. We have to get into rhythm right from the start, darling, or it will be too late."

As soon as the pistol fires we trot forward. Mum whispers in my ear—

"One-two, one-two, one-two."

We're sure-footed, in perfect time. The judge points at us, "First!" We each have a blue ribbon pinned on our shirts.

Next we line up for the egg and spoon race.

"Cath, you must stay calm. If you get too excited you'll drop the egg. Don't look at the ground and don't pay attention to anyone else around you."

Another blue ribbon for my mother and me.

I enter every track-and-field race. Left-foot, right-foot, left-foot—jump! Left-foot, right-foot, left-foot—jump! Sometimes I knock a hurdle down and have cuts and scrapes all over my legs. One of the other mothers is horrified.

"Just look at your legs! What a tomboy you are."

My mother is on the sidelines watching me in all the races.

"That was quite a day, love! I'm so proud of you."

"I'm not like a boy, am I? Sylvia's mum says I'm a tomboy."

"Oh no, you're perfect the way you are, just perfect. She's just jealous because she's got such a boring daughter who never wins anything."

I get to pick out a free gift at one of the stalls that is set up at the edge of the playing field and I choose a bottle of Pine-Sol because it smells like the woods. For the rest of my life I choose Pine-Sol because it smells like the woods and reminds me of the sunny day my mother and I won blue ribbons.

I don't remember what happened to little Hughie. I don't remember how he died, do you?"

I freeze.

After my mother gets sick she only asks about my brother this once.

"Hughie died . . . he died in an accident. A long time ago."

"Isn't it funny, but I don't remember how he died."

"He died in an accident, very peacefully."

"There was a boy at the funeral who called to say he was coming out of the haze. Did it have something to do with the days of our sorrow?"

"I don't . . . yes, I think so."

"I thought I had that right."

"Quick—look at that jay trying to land on the feeder!"

"Oh, isn't he lovely? The big brute."

I tack up orange, yellow, and green neon signs in my mother's home and write messages to her using a thick black felt pen.

> Mum, this is your very own home.
> You will never have to leave here.
> You are home!

When she starts getting anxious going to bed, anxious waking up, I record tapes for her caregiver to play first thing in the morning—

"Good morning, Mum. You are safe and sound in your own home. Time for breakfast! I'll be over to see you this morning."

Last thing at night—

"Time for sleep, Mum. Everything is in order. I will be over in the morning. You are in your very own bedroom with all your wonderful paintings around you. You will always be able to stay in your own home."

All day long for months, for years, we talk about home.

"I thought—why do I not go back where I came from, despite the fact that you're here and you came for me?"

"Wouldn't you rather stay here, in your own home?"

"I don't know. . . . I haven't got a moral yet. Still thinking about it. I'm thinking about any restrictions on going back home or coming here. I want to know what they are. I own this one? I don't, I don't own these others? But I understood I did."

"Well, I think you only own one home unless you've become a real estate baron."

"Oh no no no, don't be a smart-ass. But this is in my name?"

"It sure is, so don't you think it would be better to just stay put?"

"That's what I'm figuring. But I'm trying to figure this out, you see. If I'm not here, it's not my house."

I take her hand.

"What are you doing?"

"I'm just holding your hand."

"That's mine!"

"I know it is, Mum. This is your home and you can stay here forever, there's nowhere else you need to go."

"Who said that?"

"I'm saying that!"

"Is it my house? There must be a written thing that said I could stay here if I wished."

I show her the legal title on her property but there are too many dates, lists, words. I type up a new document:

You are the owner of the property that you live in right now. You will never have to move. You may stay in this home forever and it is fully paid for. Congratulations!

—The Land Titles Office June 2004

"What nonsense, it's not June. It must be forged."

I come back with a new document, no date.

"Nothing has to be done then? I like a deal to be cut and dried. We'll leave it for a day."

"Yes. Let's leave it for a day, now that we're all set."

"I'm sorry I'm such a bugger, Cath. I'm at such a loss in my affairs and what I owe and you know, it's amazing. I'm not as dumb as I seem. I know nothing."

"What do you mean?"

"I'm wanting this and wanting that and wanting that all the time."

"I don't notice that about you."

"Well, I haven't any tears if that's what you're wondering. I don't know, I just don't know. This is my home, I stay here?"

"Yes."

"Oh, I go backwards now. Gran and Grampy aren't coming back?"

"No, they're . . . they're in Heaven."

"Don't cry, darling. Don't cry. Well, we'll have another talk sometime. Glad to start it off bravely."

I remember how my brother died.

Early August. That last weary hour before darkness. I remember what happened two months before my mother is to remarry and we're to get our new father. Two months before our move to the city.

My brother is thirteen. I'm ten.

Boys yelling, car doors slamming, speeding away tire-screeching. A knock at the door. My brother's friend is standing there, crying. At first I think he's kidding and start to laugh but then I see the tears rolling down his face. I've never seen a big boy cry, it must be something really bad.

"Hughie's hurt. Somebody beat him up. He won't wake up."

Mum and Gran run out the door.

"Stay here, Cath."

"I want to come with you, Mum. Mum?"

She rushes out, I follow. A little way down the road there's a group of people looking at something lying in the grass by the side of the road.

———

My brother.

He's lying on his back. One of his shoes is missing and I want to go look for it because he wouldn't like that. His face is all bloody and his mouth is full of throw-up. Is he asleep?

"Mum? Mum? Is Hughie sick? How can he breathe like that?"

My mother is kneeling beside him but I can't hear what she's saying.

"Mummy? You should wake Hughie up. Why won't Hughie wake up?"

"Go back inside the house, love. Oh please, Cath, go back inside."

It's getting dark. I don't know what to do. What should I do? My gran's crying. Everybody's crying. I don't know what's going on. Why is nobody doing anything? Mum stays beside my brother and holds his hand but he wouldn't let her do that if he was awake. I'm cold. The gravel hurts my bare feet.

The police come. An ambulance. Our doctor.

What are the police doing here? Their big black car is parked at the side of the road and the red light is flashing around and around. I wish they'd turn it off because people are getting out of their cars to see what's going on and I don't want anyone staring at my brother. I watch the policeman talking to my mum. Is she in trouble? People are whispering.

"They know who did it. They're going after him right now."

Who are they talking about? What did he do? I can't stop shaking. I think I'm going to be sick. A grown-up tries to take my hand.

"Come on, dear. Let's go back inside."

"No! I'm staying here with my brother."

"Other people are with him, it's all right."

I know it isn't.

I go back inside. Sit at the kitchen table. My brother's frayed tartan bedroom slippers are leaning against my gum boots in the utility room. One of the soles is dangling loose.

Car doors slam. Motors start. Then—nothing. My mum comes back in. Her hands are shaking.

"Hughie's gone. He died, Cath. Our Hughie's gone."

"Gone where? What? Oh no. Please, Mum, no."

That night my mum talks on the phone to the man who's going to be her new husband and our new father. He's away on business. She turns her back, whispering sobs into the phone.

"Hughie's been killed. I don't know—a boy—yes, drunk—much older—pulled over— started a fight— he was after Hughie's friend, but—"

I close my eyes.

"Please God please God please God I promise to be a better nicer kinder person if only it isn't true. Please God don't let Hughie be dead please God please please please."

My grandmother and I cry all night long and the next day and the next and the next but after that first night my mother never cries about my brother in front of me again.

For the rest of the summer I spend a lot of time in the backyard. I find a new hiding place beside the fence and have to crawl through thorny blackberry bushes to get in and out. I lie on the long soft grass and watch the clouds and once I see a train cloud float by. Gran says train clouds take children to Heaven and I wonder if my brother Hughie's on that train.

When Mum or Gran calls I answer right away.
  "I'm here, I'm right here! Coming!"

One day I go to my new hiding place but there are big skinny spiders everywhere so I don't go there anymore.

My friends want me to go bike riding but I don't feel like it.

Sometimes I walk over to the neighbors' but I never walk on the side of the road where my brother died. I'm afraid I might see something. Late at night I lie in bed and listen to frog-croaking and cricket-chirping and wonder if the boy who killed my brother will be back.

My parents spend their weekend honeymoon at a local resort that has an indoor pool and horseback riding. They take me with them. A relative tells me what a lucky girl I am.

"Most stepfathers wouldn't take a child along on a honeymoon."

My new dad buys me a white shirt with a red fringe and two brown horses on the front. We have dinner in the hotel restaurant every night and my father always lets me order a Shirley Temple. There's a big dance floor and all the tables have white cloths and candles. The bandleader announces that my parents just got married. They play "The Hawaiian Wedding Song" and make them get up and dance all by themselves and everyone claps.

> *Now that we are one*
> *Clouds won't hide the sun*
> *Blue skies of Hawaii smile*
> *On this, our wedding day*
> *I do love you with all my heart.*

———

My father holds my mother close and when the dance is over he takes her elbow and leads her back to the table. Pulling out her chair, he smiles.

"Good, good, good. I'm a lucky man."

Mum and I take turns dancing with him and when it's my turn we circle around the room—slow, slow, quick-quick. He squeezes my hand really tight and out of the corner of my eye I see his chin sticking out and watch the other dancers get out of his way.

My dad starts the paperwork to adopt me. I want the same name my mother and father have. A new name. A social worker comes to see me and asks if there's any reason I don't want to be adopted by my new father. There isn't.

After my mum remarries I want to stay behind at my island school and board for a year. We pack my royal blue metal trunk.

"Now love, I'm only a ferry ride away and I'll be over to see you in only two weeks."

My mother packs my brand new riding boots and English jodhpurs.

"Oh please can I try my boots on just once more? I can't wait to see all my friends again and find out what horses I'll ride this year. Do you think they'll let me ride Sammy, Mum? Do you?"

"Last time, Cath, and then we have to pack them away. Won't it be fun to open your trunk with all these lovely things inside?"

"Mum, Hughie gave me a really nice smile the night he died, I mean—before he went out. He did, Mum."

"Did he, darling? He loved you very much."

She writes to me every week.

September 12, 1963

My darling,
I so hope you are having fun with all your friends and I know you are happy at your lovely school. Grade Six already! Mummy is very happy here. I tidied up a little today and did some shopping then I spoke to quite a few friends on the phone and then got dinner, so it was lovely to be just a plain housewife again. Uncle Hugh dropped in and had tea with me, so it was like playing house. Be a good girl and try hard at school, dear. We will be over for your birthday. Dad sends his love and lots and lots from your loving Mum. xoxox

Sometimes they come over for the weekend and we stay in a motel. They always bring me presents and for my birthday I get a camera so I can take pictures of all my favorite horses.

"Dad and I are proud of you for doing so well in school and making all the teams!"

My new dad is happy.

"Gosh, that's right. Good for you!"

———

57

Once a year our headmistress has each class of boarders over for tea with real china cups and saucers and we get all dressed up. She puts our names at each place setting and I lie awake all night hoping she'll sit me beside her. She makes little cucumber sandwiches with the crusts cut off, scones with homemade strawberry jam, and Spotted Dog with cream and warm syrup.

"You know, girls, my mother taught me how to make Spotted Dog. She'd say to me, 'Mind, my lovey, that you be sure to cut a deep cross in the round of dough, to let the fairies out.'"

We sit in her little home and listen to stories about her childhood in Ireland and how she came to be a teacher and headmistress.

"Now girls, you can accomplish anything you want, you only need to believe in yourselves. The best life is one in which you do good things for other people and for the world in which you live."

When I get back to the dorm I write down everything she has said.

One day my friends and I climb the old oak tree to watch the seniors play in the grass hockey finals.

"Did your brother really die?"

Everyone stops talking. I'm embarrassed and don't know what to say.

"Um, this summer he—"

The girl who asks leans over and pushes me off my branch. I fall, catching my skirt on a lower limb and dangle upside down until I can get hold of another branch and climb to the ground. I'm mad she caught me off guard. Mad I fell.

Every day I pretend my brother stands on the gym roof waving and waving.

"I'm coming, Cath! I'm coming."

The following year I leave my island school and move to the city to board at a different school twenty minutes from where my parents live.

"It will be wonderful to have you so much closer, love."

A big-city boarding school where there are no Friday night movies with two scoops of ice cream, no tree climbing, no riding lessons or racing to the stables on cold dark winter mornings—the stalls fragrant with oats, leather, liniment, and horse. No weekend passes home.

Anxiety begins to set up house inside my mother's head. She calls every hour, forgets we've just spoken. Her signature ring—insistent, startling, urgent. I run to catch her calls.

"Where are you, love? I've called and called."

"I'm fine. I was at the dentist's, remember?"

"Oh, but I read in the paper that we should take a second look and feel good about it. Did you have anywhere to go with my mind?"

"What? No, I thought I'd leave it right where it is. Yes, that's safer, isn't it?"

"But where did you put all that information?"

"In my head."

"Oh dear."

"It doesn't matter, does it?"

"Not unless a car is coming."

I sign up for ballroom and Latin dance classes. I want to move to music and get out of my head. Get my mother out of my head. I go to all the group and practice parties but I don't tell anyone about her.

The cha-cha—perky and playful, 1-2-3, 4 & 1, 2-3 . . . but I'm frantic, feral.

"We want some of what you're on. You always look like you're having so much fun!"

Fun? Can't you hear me crying in the bathroom? My mother is . . . I can barely get out of bed to come here, you stupid goddamn idiots!

I would never say.

"The Latin dances really suit you. You have so much energy."

Shut up shut up shut up.

I dance nine hours a week at the studio and practice at home and at the gym. A beginning pain creeps into my left hip.

Sinatra croons Irving Berlin, a slow waltz.

I'm just the words, looking for the tune,
Reaching for the moon and you . . .

1-2-3, 2-2-3, 3-2-3, 4-2-3 . . .

I close my eyes. Imagine seabirds riding wind currents over a slate-gray wintry sea.

5-2-3, 6-2-3 . . .

I call my mother to say good night before I leave the dance studio.

"I don't have to be personable all the time, do I, Mum?"

"Well, on a personal basis . . . yes, I think you do."

"Oh dear. Well, I'll call you in the morning."

"Nighty-night, Hughie Boy. Oh, but aren't you coming over?"

"Hughie? Um . . . I'm at, I just got into bed. Is something wrong?"

"I don't know that I want to tell you anything or end up saying anything because as long as I've known when you've asked me anything and I've answered you very nicely, I've got a real boo."

"A real what?"

"Boo, boom. I don't think you took it seriously at all. I think it was a big laugh. When you were small-ish and growing up and even now I think you would say, 'What do you think of that man, Mum?' and I would say, 'I think he's lovely.' And then you would say, 'Lovely?'"

"Oh, I—"

"Yeah. No, no, no."

"I'm sorry . . . I'll try to be more careful."

"Well I don't know because I don't know, I don't know you any longer."

I'm sick of myself. Sick of not being strong enough to handle sorrow. My mother's. Mine.

Sick of my bed, I move to the couch in front of the fire and close the blinds. My cat lands beside me softly, like a bird. I nuzzle into his warm belly soothed by his earthy scent. He swats at me. Moves away.

Late into the night the radio keeps me company. A talk show, jazz, two Chinese-language stations, a preacher. I listen carefully. Wait for someone to tell me what to do.

I don't know where my will is, have I made a will? I must make a will."

"You already have a will. Your lawyer has the original, remember?"

"I have not made a will. You'll have to call my lawyer."

I show her a copy of her will.

"That's not mine."

"Yes it is, see where you've signed it?"

"That's not my signature."

"Oh, I'm all mixed up, Mum. Let's just change the subject, it's getting irritating."

"It was from the word go."

"Would you like a cup of tea?"

"Oh how lovely. Where is my will? Did you sign this one?"

"No! Oh gee, I don't know, I'm going to go crazy in a minute! I think I'll go home now, I'm just so tired and this place it's . . . it's just too crazy here today."

"It wasn't crazy before you got here."

I stay.

"You're getting pretty funny, aren't you, Mum?"

"Do you mean funny queer?"
"No, I mean funny amusing."
"Oh, that's good."
"It's a fine line though, isn't it?"
"It is with me."

I start seeing a family therapist who works with midlife children caring for aging parents. She knows how my mother and I spend our days, hours, minutes.

She has a cat.

I tell her I can't breathe with all the worry sitting on my chest. She gets the cat, plops her down beside me. Sometimes I take my writing over, read out my pencil-scratchings—mother, boarding school, men. She teases out essence, points of view.

We watch my dance videos—slow, slow, quick-quick, slow.

"You describe the experience of looking after your mother in some of the same ways you talk about dance."

I am choreographing a dance for my mother and me.

At my new boarding school I run for my mother's calls every Wednesday night for six years. She's allowed to call me once a week, but if the line's busy or it's after lights-out I won't be able to talk to her. I can't call her back because we're not allowed to make telephone calls without written permission. Every week I wait in line to see the assistant headmistress.

Wednesday, 16th Sept. 1964

May I please have permission to call home?

Thank you.
Cathie

Sometimes she says no. "You've already called home this week, you know the rules."

I don't want anyone to see me crying so I hide in the bathroom. At night I lie in bed and pretend my new dad phones the school.

"Cathie is going to be a day girl from now on. She'll be living at home with us."

I write Mum at least once a week and every day after school I rush over to the main residence to wait for mail call.

November 15, 1964

My Dear Cath,

It was wonderful to see you on Saturday, love. Didn't we have fun shopping? I'm so glad that you liked your new blouse and I'm thrilled with my hat. It's just the thing for the luncheon Dad and I are going to in London! Now that exams are just around the corner you'll have to get right down to studying, darling. Grade Seven is an important year! Then you will be home for Christmas, and that will be wonderful. I know Gran can hardly wait as well. We'll have a lot of fun. I'd better run, love, as I have shopping to do for dinner and it's nearly four o'clock! I will call Wednesday. Always remember that your Mum loves you very much, Cath.
P.S. The $1.00 is from Dad!

Only the grade twelves are allowed to walk up to the local shops after school for an hour on their own. Except for holidays, long weekends, and Saturdays from eleven to eight, boarders aren't allowed to stay out overnight or leave the school grounds. Most live too far away to go home, and even though my parents live only twenty minutes from the school I'm not allowed to go home for the weekend. We all have to do the same thing.

Saturdays. Eleven to eight. Not Sundays, Sundays are for church. A yellow school bus takes us downtown to a church ten minutes from where my parents live. We line up on the street two-by-two in our white woolen berets and white gloves, navy blue blazers and tartan skirts, navy kneesocks and black oxfords—a spectacle for bystanders, tourists, churchgoers.

The church is dark, soothing. I close my eyes, breathe in oak, sandalwood, candle wax, and watch the light flicker through stained glass windows in flashes of crimson and gold. My favorite pane is St. Francis of Assisi standing under a bright blue sky, a fawn at his side, a lark on his shoulder. I love singing hymns and know the words to most of them. Hate it when they don't play my favorites, "All Things Bright and Beautiful," "Fairest Lord Jesus," "St. Patrick's Breastplate." We all adore our minister whose Irish lilt lulls and inspires, but my last prayer is always a plea.

"Please God, maybe you could figure a way for me to be at home. I really want to go home and be with my mum. Please God."

During the week we have morning prayers in the gym and evening prayers in the residence. I spend a lot of time talking to God, apologizing.

"I'm sorry for fooling around in math class, Lord, and for making my history teacher mad and I'm sorry for being so mean to my roommate but sometimes I just hate her so much, hate her stupid straight blonde hair and that she's so pretty."

That I'm not.

Daygirls are sent to good private schools by well-to-do-parents who were sent to the same good private schools. Boarders are girls from other countries whose parents want them to have a better education, girls from small communities with mediocre schools, from logging towns, remote islands, broken homes. Some are girls who have been getting into trouble or are headed for trouble. Daughters of busy stepfathers.

Some daygirls ignore boarders, some boarders resent daygirls and think they're snobs. Someone says that my father's name, though respected, is not "old money." That he's a self-made man and makes business, not social liaisons. I like this about my father.

Over Christmas and summer holidays boarders go home. Many daygirls leave for sunny holidays and vacation homes and no one lives downtown where we live. Our two-bedroom rented apartment, close to my father's downtown office, caters to singles and old people, not to parents with one young teenager. Mum says that one of Dad's business partners asked him why he doesn't buy a house so I could live at home.

"Oh, Mum, really? What did he say?"

"Nothing. I thought he might. . . . He didn't say anything, love."

Everybody says my new father is an important businessman and that he's worked hard for his money. My mother doesn't have to work anymore and she signs up for flower arranging and sewing classes at the local community center.

"The florist says I'm the most creative student he's ever had—can you believe it, Cath?"

My father buys her an expensive sewing machine. She clips a dress pattern out of "The Sewing Corner" in the newspaper and makes an emerald silk dress to wear to an international trade luncheon with my father. He is very proud of her.

"Gosh sakes, you look wonderful. Good, good, good."

She joins the local orchid society and learns how to measure air humidity with a hygrometer. There are orchids and African violets in pretty green and pink china pots all over the apartment. During the week, she visits nurseries and plant stores and sometimes her brother, Hugh, takes the afternoon off from work and goes with her. They drive for hours through farmland, stopping by the river to eat Cheez Whiz sandwiches and drink coffee from a thermos. They sit and watch tugboats pressing into the sides of barges, herding.

My grandmother has moved from her island home to an apartment two blocks from ours. She doesn't want to live in the country anymore. My stepfather pays for her rent and food and my mother takes her to the grocery store, the bank, her medical appointments, and uses her own housekeeping money to buy her clothes. Every day there is something she has to do for my grandmother.

"I hardly have anything left over at the end of the month, Cath."

"Can't you ask Dad for more money?"

"Oh no, love. He wouldn't like that."

I visit my gran when I'm home from school on Saturdays and every day during the holidays.

"Gran, remember that time Hughie and I put all those cedar branches in the garage and Mum couldn't park the car?"

"Please don't mention his name, pet. I just can't bear it . . ."

During our walks in the park she points out her favorite plants with her wooden cane—the old-fashioned roses, a clematis, the scented hybrid rhododendron. Late afternoons we have tea and gingersnaps and sometimes for a treat she'll make me coconut macaroons or Scotch scones.

"What a pity Mum and Dad have to go out tonight and you have to go back to school early. Still, they usually do, don't they? I don't know why you have to go to that awful school. I wish you could live here with me, but I'm too old for all that now."

Every morning and evening we walk three long blocks back and forth from the boarding annex to the main school. I board with girls from all over the province, the country, the world. I never see anyone cry but I hear crying in the middle of the night.

We walk two by two. No talking allowed with the girls in front or behind. Two matrons escort us, one leads the front of the line, one brings up the back. I'm always in trouble for fooling around, for minor pranks. The head matron marches up and down the line—scolding, picking, nagging.

"Catherine, face the front."

"Catherine, if I find you talking to the girls behind one more time I'll see you miss your hockey game."

She makes a "teh-teh" sound between each word accompanied by a constant humming. Her eyes dart up and down the line as she flicks her thumb against each of her fingers beginning with her index finger and running down to her baby finger and back, over and over. She wakes us every morning ringing an iron bell at the foot of our beds. She doesn't like me,

I don't know why. One night she slaps me across the face, leaving a crimson imprint on my cheek. The other girls stare in silence and horror, nobody knows what to do.

"One of the matrons hit me across the face, Mum. Can you come and get me? Please Dad, don't make me stay here anymore."

I never say.

The school awards points for good grades, team participation, punctuality, tidiness, and for general helpfulness, but there are no points awarded for tomfoolery or making the other girls laugh. My grades drop from A to C, and I'm moved into the stupid class. My report cards always say the same thing. *Catherine spends far too much time entertaining the other girls and wasting precious classroom time. She will need to settle down and apply herself if she is to do well.*

If we step out of line—littering, uniform infractions, late homework—we have to stand outside the headmistress's office so everyone walking by can see we've done something wrong, but we all think this is funny. Sometimes we're sent to the infirmary for a few hours of isolation but the nurse is nice and there's a big window looking out over the garden and tennis courts. We lose phone and going-home privileges for

big things like lying, cheating, or talking back. On
the big things, I behave.

Our headmistress is short, stout, and plain. Clever.
Meant for an earlier time, she lacks the stomach to
guide us through the sixties, but when she reads Yeats
she closes her eyes and rocks back and forth, a thin
private smile etched across her face.

> *How many loved your moments of glad grace,*
> *And loved your beauty with love false or true;*
> *But one man loved the pilgrim soul in you . . .*

Some girls make fun of her. Mostly, I don't.

M y father buys four lots of waterfront up the coast and has a house built. He knows how much my mother loves the sea.

"You're to design it yourself. Anything you want— just as long as I get my sauna. And you're to have your boat."

The first of my mother's three boats is a blue-and-white 16-footer with a single 60-horsepower engine. Her second boat, orange, is a 160-horsepower inboard-outboard with sleeper beds for overnight fishing trips. Her third and last boat is a 28-foot sports fisher with double 250-horsepower inboard engines, VHF/CB radio, depth sounder, and an electric anchor. The cabin has a galley, a head, and room to sleep four.

"I never should have bought the *Rain Bird*, love. It was too much boat for me."

She signs up for the Canadian Power and Sail Squadrons course and studies boating safety and operation, compass readings, marine rules, trip planning, weather, and navigation. At graduation she receives a badge with the squadron crest—a red maple leaf set against a blue-and-white-striped flag bordered by a gold-braided ship's wheel, with a matching flag to fly on the stern of her boat. She takes a second course in advanced navigation and late into the night deciphers the language of the sea, analyzing marine charts with symbols indicating navigational aids for lighthouses, beacons, buoys, channels, dangerous rocks, and speed limits.

"Cath, when you're coming into the harbor you must always keep the red light on your right. If you steer to the right of it you'll hit land. Here's how you remember it, love: red—right—returning."

My father is very proud of my mother.

"I don't know how you do it."

Uncle Hugh and his family sometimes visit and in the evenings my cousins and I play with the Ouija board, my aunt knits, and my father sits silently with his *Financial Post*, the local and national newspapers, and company reports. My uncle helps my mother practice her marine knots.

"Jo, the two half-hitch is quick to tie and easy to undo so we can use it for mooring, and I like the bowline because it doesn't jam or slip. Remember when we used to tie all these as kids?"

"You boys tied them, Hugh, I never did. I'm never going to get this right, I'm so slow!"

"Come on, kid, let's do them all again."

By the end of the course all her knots are perfect.

My mother and uncle never tell us where they're going fishing in the morning. They choose a spot based on the weather, tides, their instincts, and tips from the bait vendors. All day long they sit together, my mother and her brother, watching their lines and the sea. Her brother has taught her everything she knows about fishing. He's her favorite fishing partner. Her favorite everything.

Often it's just the three of us up at our home by the sea.

My father and I make bad fishing companions. My father is restless, and all I want to do is lie on the deck, reading. Mostly, my mother fishes alone.

She sits in her boat from early morning until late afternoon. When she gets a bite she grabs the rod and pulls up hard, sets the hook then reels in, lets it run, reels in, lets it run, keeping her rod tip up and the line tight until the fish is too tired to fight anymore. She nets it, lifts it over the gunnel, and gives it a quick, hard smack to the head. There are other boats about but none with a five-foot two-inch blond, suntanned woman sitting alone, fishing. Not one.

At four I start watching for her boat to come around the point. She makes a perfect landing, ties up at our dock, and gives us the thumbs-up. She hardly ever gets skunked. Slipping her fingers inside the gills she holds up her fish and my father shouts down from the deck. "Oh gosh, salmon for dinner!"

Using the fish table her brother built for her she makes a deep cut at the back of the neck and slices off the head then turns the fish on its back, cuts down the length from vent to neck, and splits the belly wide open. Pulling out the guts and heart she opens up the stomach.

"There's my bait, you greedy thing!"

She slices open the kidney, scraping clean the small white sac of jelly-like blood that runs along the spine. Flocks of screeching seagulls circle the wharf, dive-bombing for the bloody head and entrails she tosses them. By the time she climbs up the steep path to the house she's out of breath, smiling.

"It was like glass out there. Oh boy, what a day . . ."

My father turns on the 8:00 a.m. news before he gets out of bed, resting the radio on his chest as he waits for the stock market report. During the day he carries his radio in his back pocket so he can listen to the hourly news. He spends his day chopping wood, slashing back salal, and managing his side of the garden. His dahlias and gladioli, which he stakes and ties with the little bits of string he keeps in his pocket, stand tall and vibrant. He carries his pruning shears with him all day long— clipping, trimming, cutting back. Nothing on my father's side of the garden is allowed to wander or grow wild.

At noon my dad and I sit together for cottage cheese, fruit salad, and toast. During the war he earned the nickname Jammy, always hoping he'd be sent jam in a care package. I bring a jar to the table.

"Here you go, Jammy!"

At three thirty I turn on the sauna and by four he is happily sweating and scrubbing in his cedar-scented sanctuary. Later, he lies on his bed in his blue tartan housecoat, exercising his fingers. I watch him from the bedroom door, his lips are moving but I can't hear what he is saying.

"What are you doing, Dad?"

"Oh, I'm just giving myself a little pep talk, lovey. Thinking about my jam, and how lucky I am to have you and Mummy, and this beautiful home. Gosh, it's wonderful!"

First thing in the morning I tie an apron around my waist, and all day long I measure, mix, and bake. My mother has taught me the secret to making perfect pastry.

"Now listen, love, each ingredient must be cold and your measurements have to be accurate. Handle the mixture as little and lightly as possible and don't use too much water. The oven needs to be exactly the right temperature."

I mix together flour, salt, baking powder, then cut in the shortening with my grandmother's red-handled pastry cutter. After adding in cold water a little at a time, I rub a light coat of flour on my hands, roll the dough into a ball, wrap it in wax paper, and set it to rest in the fridge for an hour. I wash each dish as I go along.

"It's so much nicer not having a mess at the end, isn't it, Cath?"

Rolling the pastry from the center out I fold the dough in half and lay it over the plate, using a fork to press a pattern around the edge.

I tell my father I'm going for a quick swim and dive into the cold briny darkness, washing off sweat and sticky pieces of dough. Closing my eyes against the piercing reflection of the late afternoon sun I breathe in the salty scent of low tide as the waves rock me back and forth.

After dinner my mother plays the piano. Sometimes I talk my dad into singing one of his old favorites.

More than the greatest love the world
*   has known,*
This is the love I give to you alone.

He claps his hands and laughs, embarrassed. I beg
my mother to play "My Little Corner of the World"
and usually miss the A-flat but she shouts above the
music, nodding her head.

"Just keep going, love. Come on, keep going!"

At the end of our day my father and I praise my
mother for the salmon she's caught and my parents
thank me for the meal I've set before them. In the
evening, we walk through the garden and my mother
and I admire my father's gladioli.

Each of us weaves through our day taken up with
the things we love.

S mall talk at the dance studio.
"Hi there how are you oh you know too busy gee isn't the weather awful I hate this rain Mexico sounds good yeah I know what you mean what a drag my shoulder's killing me I've just got to get back to the gym I'm so fat call me!"

Nothing talk.

"Hello," says a man at the studio. I start to cry.

"I can't think today and I don't want to hear 'Hi there! How are you?' one more stupid goddamn time!"

"Come, sit."

"I'm going to kill the next person who says that."

He stands beside me, his hand lightly on my shoulder. Doesn't talk.

Women gather on the edges of the dance floor.

"Too many beginners tonight."

"No one's asked me to dance, I'm leaving."

"Only the young girls get asked to dance."

———

I hide in the bathroom, pretend allergies, until the beginning notes of an Argentine tango draw me back into the studio. I wrap my arm around a man's back, close my eyes, and settle . . . like a rider sinking down into the sway of a horse's back.

My mother thinks she's being poisoned. I type up instructions and ask her doctor to sign them.

<u>Doctor's Orders for Mrs. B.</u>
1. In order to strengthen your legs I want you to take the blue pill once a day.
2. Drink one glass of prune juice every morning.
3. Drink one glass of the orange drink, Metamucil, half an hour after meals. This will keep food moving down in a regular manner.
4. You may take the red pill, Tylenol, two or three times a day for aches and pains.

This is a very good routine for you, Mrs. B., and important for your health. I'm really pleased with your progress, you are doing a great job.

At the pharmacy I renew prescriptions: diuretics, antibiotics. Try new ones: Aricept, Paxil, Seroquel, L-DOPA. Re-stock supplies: Tylenol, Metamucil, Telpha pads, Polysporin, peroxide, Gravol, Maalox, Senokot, Magnolax, Imodium, Tums. I ask the pharmacist for advice.

"If someone you love is old and suffering and you look after them for years and years, how do you not go crazy?"

"Most people put them in a home. Visit once a month."

At the home-care store I watch people move from shelf to shelf looking for answers. Utensil holders, jar openers, elastic laces, extra-long shoehorn, under-knee support pillow, air cushion ring, shower chair, bath railings, body cleansers, commode, raised toilet seat, transfer devices, cane, walker, wheelchair, waterproof bedding, electric bed lift, adult diapers, cleansing cloths, hospital bed.

Our days, weeks, months taken up with visits to the doctor, the pharmacy, the hospital. Four years of infections, falls, arthritis, tests, procedures, removal of cataracts and skin cancers, brain scans, X-rays. The gerontology consult. Getting in and out of the car.

Find handicap parking please God please God. Lift wheelchair out of the trunk open passenger door lift Mum out help her stand shift to wheelchair lift legs onto foot pedals oh careful push wheelchair up steep incline grind teeth against jabs in left hip go to appointment don't cry don't cry wheel back to car lift her out of the wheelchair into car clip seatbelt kiss forehead lift wheelchair into trunk left hip left hip drive to mall for lunch lift wheelchair out of the trunk. In and out.

Three concrete planters sit outside the main hospital entrance, filled with earth, dead plants, and cigarette butts.

"Can't they at least clean up this goddamn mess?"

"Oh you mustn't, love. What a shame though, such a nice shady spot for impatiens."

The gerontologist is going to figure out what's wrong with my mother's mind and tell me what I already know. She has a long list of questions for her.

"Good morning. Is this your daughter?"

"Yes."

"Do you have any other children?"

"No."

When my mother is asked to write her name on a piece of paper her signature is tiny, scratchy, unfamiliar. The doctor asks her to draw a clock and set the time to eleven thirty. She tells her to count backward from one hundred, in sevens. The questions go on and on.

"What is your name? Can you write your name down for me? Where are we right now? What is your address? Where were you born? Who's our premier? How would you get home from here?"

I'm answering each question in my head, my underarms are soaked—I can't remember the name of our premier. My mother doesn't know her address or where we are. The doctor asks me to leave so she can talk with my mother alone. Her tone dismissive. We never see her again.

During the next visit to my doctor's I tell her she must never ask me to count backward in sevens and that she has to write this down in my chart.

"Why not?"

"I can't even do it now!"

The plastic surgeon who removes skin lesions from her face has no kind words for my mother. I watch as he roughly inserts the needle into her thin, tender skin. She never complains. I scream at him in my head—*you stupid jerk I hate you!* I think I'm going to faint and have to leave the room. Hospital staff breeze by laughing and chatting on their way to the cafeteria.

Back home, we sit and discuss the day.

"You're so brave, Mum. What do you think courageous means?"

"Well, courageous means brave in front of other people."

"I think it means brave alone, too."

"Oh, that's what I want. I still want to keep that."

"Which do you like better, love or hate?"

"Hate."

"Because?"

"This is a very difficult question as so many people are vanished into the hate business."

We munch on biscuits.

"I was wondering about the seats in the church . . . wondering if you've banked any."

"What? Um . . . yes, we have lots banked. All up to date."

"Oh good."

"Do you think you're a good listener?"

"No, I don't think so."

"What makes you say that?"

"I don't think I am a good listener. I don't like to get around to people who are talking shop or talking about trips they've been on but they say everybody is laughing a lot. I'm even sitting there thinking—oh God will they ever, will it ever end? So I have to be honest and say no, I'm not really very interested."

"Which do you like better, fish or birds?"

"Fish."

"Because?"

"May I make that a little bit noisy?"
"Please do."
My mother gestures, lets out her fishing line.
"Because they're easier for every man to catch."

When she's not away on a business trip with my father, my mother picks me up from boarding school every Saturday at eleven o'clock. The best part is just before I see her new blue Mustang turning into the drive. Before I start counting how many hours I have left.

<u>Eleven o'clock</u>

We drive straight downtown and spend the whole day together. For lunch we go to our favorite department store and I have macaroni and cheese, green peas, and cherry Jell-O with a dollop of whipped cream on top. I squish the red up against the roof of my mouth until it turns to liquid then swallow it, like medicine. My mother always buys me nylons or kneesocks and something special, a blouse, shoes, or the latest Beatles album. Sometimes we walk down to Millar and Coe to look at the china.

"I'm buying Willow Pattern when I get married. Just like Gran's."

"Wouldn't that be lovely? Do you remember the rhyme about the pattern? Gran said it was very old and probably made up by a scullery maid in England,

many years ago. She used to recite it to me when I
was just a little girl—

> *Two pigeons flying high,*
> *Chinese vessels sailing by,*
> *Weeping willows hanging o'er*
> *Bridge with three men, if not four,*
> *Chinese Temple, there it stands,*
> *Seems to take up all the land,*
> *Apple trees with apples on*
> *A pretty fence to end my song."*

One Saturday we visit an old friend of my mother's
for tea. She asks me to help her in the kitchen.

"Now dear, it's best if you don't talk about your
brother to your mum. It's just too upsetting for her.
You understand, don't you, dear?"

We go back into the living room with tea and toast-
ed crumpets.

"A new school and a new father? He's very well
known in the business community, you know. Aren't
you the lucky girl?"

A new father. A provider of money (thank you) private school (thank you) nice clothes (thank you) a
vacation home, ski lessons, tennis lessons (thank
you), anything necessary and many things that were

not. Thank you. A new father who doesn't come to the school plays I'm in, Sports Day, the annual debate I won (traveling) (meetings) (traveling), misses the annual Father-Daughter Dinners (International Trade Fair), away for most of my birthdays (Canadian Chamber of Commerce).

Three o'clock
At home we have a cup of tea and Mum's homemade chocolate chip cookies. Sometimes she helps me memorize poems for my English class.

"Stand tall, love, and lift your head up so I can hear you. Go slowly, one line at a time until you are sure you know each line before you move on to the next one. Picture each word. It's always easier to remember the lines when you understand the story."

I start packing while my mother bakes me brownies with walnuts in them to take back to school. After they're cool she cuts them into squares, wraps them in wax paper and foil, then layers them neatly inside a square tin. At school I hide them under my bed and eat them when no one's looking.

Four o'clock
My father comes home from his Saturday at the office and announces himself with his customary

two-note whistle. I wish he would come home later so I could have more time alone with Mum. He kisses my mother then walks down the hall to their bedroom. He sits on the woven chair beside the bed, takes his shoes and socks off and puts on clean socks and his bedroom slippers.

"My feet take care of me and I take care of my feet!"

On his way down to the living room he pops his head into the den.

"Mummy's cooking a good dinner!"

Settled on the couch he reads his newspapers and business magazines and listens to the five o'clock news. We always have dinner on TV tables in the den so he can watch the six o'clock news. After dinner he goes back to his papers.

I wish just Mum would take me back to school, but my father usually insists on driving. I sit in the front between my parents, holding back tears.

She comes into the residence to sign me back in and then is gone.

My father and I never do anything alone. I don't know what to talk about. I just want to be alone with my mum all the time.

"You two always pair up."

I know my mother would like it if I made more effort with my father but I don't. I wanted a new father badly until this boarding school. I blame him for this boarding school. Blame him for everything.

G rade eleven. I call my parents.

"Guess what? I've been made a house captain!"

The headmistress announces it in front of the whole school in morning assembly and we get to go up on stage to receive our house sashes that we will wear every day over our uniforms. As house captains we are in charge of instilling enthusiasm and school loyalty. We run regular meetings and put up notices on our house bulletin boards in the hall. I can hardly wait for the day to start so I can put up inspirational quotes.

> Character cannot be developed in ease and quiet. Only through experience can the soul be strengthened, ambition inspired, and success achieved.
>
> —Helen Keller

September, grade twelve. I make prefect. We get to wear white blazers. I wanted to be head girl but am made head boarder. We are called into the headmistress's office.

"All eyes are on you, and you must be vigilant in your roles as leaders. You have added authority now and will be supervising the girls as they go about their days. But it is most important that you lead with compassion and always put the name of the school first."

Everyone says how important this will be for our future careers.

As head boarder, I help out with evening prayers and organize events. I'm to keep an eye out for the younger girls, making sure they are not left out of school activities, or feeling too homesick.

L ove? How do I get home or when I get home how do I get home?"

"Mum, you are home, see all your things around you?"

"These are my things? How did they get here? I think that girl, she was the one I found most interesting but sometimes I think she employed too much use of the wind."

"Who? Who was that?"

"Who? You're a regular customer and I'm the one that rushes in, all eyes. This is my home? Do I own it?"

"Yes, you own it and you'll always be able to stay here."

"Good, because I never want to leave here. Getting them unscrambled is an important thing—you go seven, eight, nine, which means you're pretty strong which is a good thing. And the birds, that's what they were screaming about, these little ones this morning."

"What were they saying?"

"They said, 'Stay little one, stay.' And I said, 'Okay, okay.'"

"That should settle it."

I make tea.

"Tea is a more pleasant drink. It just seems to sort of go down and settle things."

"You're my favorite person in the world."

"Favorite amongst the constipated you mean."

"How was your day?"

"Today I was down at the horse barn. It came with lots of blessings."

"Oh my . . . I love listening to you talk."

"You love what?"

"Listening to you talk."

"Oh. I thought I heard you say, I love looking into your voice."

"I love that, too."

Long weekends, Christmas holidays, spring break, summer.

I'm sick of hitting the tennis ball against the practice wall in the park, alone. Sick of watching TV. I want to go back to school. See all my friends.

My mother has started crying at the end of all our visits.

"I want to go home with you, darling."

"Oh Mum, I'll call as soon as I get home. I'm only a few blocks away."

When I lean down to kiss her good night she whispers in my ear—

"Wait, love, I'm coming with you."

She tries to stand, to get out of her wheelchair.

"But I'll be back first thing in the morning."

"Don't leave me here. Take me home, Cath."

"Mum . . ."

"Oh darling, don't cry."

"I'll stay and we'll have a visit and then it will be time for our dinner."

"I think I must have had a dream and it was all to do with the blue little thing up there, you know, the little house just for good people."

"Oh? It sounds sort of like Heaven. What do you think I should do, I mean, after you're gone?"

"Well, you may be a different person. You may be a happy person, individually prominent if I can say it that way."

"Sometimes I wonder if I took up too much of your time, too much of your life."

"Oh no, you were nifty. You were a happy machine and the only one who wiggled a tune. You know, I don't know how much longer I'm going to be here but I want you to have it."

"To have—?"

"Yes, because you're the boy and you're my favorite."

I tuck her in. Drive home. Eat two bowls of cereal. Crawl into bed. Swaddled inside flannel sheets I hunker down under heavy wool blankets and wedge a pillow tight between my thighs, rocking back and forth. Into this slipped-down place drifts the memory of a man's scent.

Long after my brother's death I go back to the place where he was killed and look for signs of him, but there is nothing.

Nothing.

I pretend he isn't dead but there's no stopping the dying of my brother. I stand by the side of the road and wonder why he had to die. Like that. Nobody knows why.

There is no why.

Mum, I'll sing the first note of a song and you try to guess what it is. Here we go—*You . . .*"

Are my sunshine, my only sunshine,
You make me happy, when skies are gray,
You'll never know dear, how much I love you.
Please don't take my sunshine away.

"Beautiful, well done."

"Thank you!"

She raises her eyebrows, shrugs coquettishly.

"You have some very interesting facial expressions lately."

"Have I?"

"How would you explain those?"

"Um, coming back to life. That's all, coming back to life."

I want to keep the words of my new poet-mother.

"I'm taping our conversations, Mum."

"Is the machine recording everything now?"

"Yes."

"That's kind of silly, isn't it?"

"No, I like listening to what you have to say."

"It's not very much, is it?"

"I think it is. Your opinions are very important to me."

"I'd have to hear them and find out how important they were."

I anchor the tape recorder between pillows on her lap.

"Why do people smoke?"

"To cast off pain and loneliness."

"Why do people drink too much?"

"Because they know it's such a relief."

"And how are you enjoying your mind these days?"

"Oh, very much, very much. I wake up in the morning and the first thing I think of is myself and then next I think of myself again and the third thing is I get my breakfast."

"In the meantime do you want to tell me how you're feeling today?"

"In the meantime, no, I don't really want to, thank you."

"You sound a little down."

"A little, maybe."

"What does sorrow look like?"

"It's a form of sadness brought about on a gray and heavy day. I've reached the ultimate of the intimate and that's the end of it."

"Oh dear . . . Let me ask you, what do you think is the ugliest thing in the world?"

"A lack of dignity. Is that the right answer?"

"Yes. Okay, what about this one: what's the worst thing a person could do to another person?"

"They could throw their sublime into the ridiculous."

"What is so scary about dying?"

"Have you ever tried it?"

"Good point."

"You know, things are going the way they're going now but you don't seem to mind."

"I love it."

"You didn't like it before very much."

"No, I guess I didn't. What is the meaning of life?"

"I don't know, I haven't seen it. What are you writing down all the time?"

"I'm writing about you and all the interesting things you say."

"But do they match?"

"I don't know."

"Don't think for a moment any of it's foolproof."

In the spring of grade twelve I am called into the head-mistress's office. The assistant head is there too and I know by the look on their faces that something is very wrong. Someone has told them that I smoked a joint once at a party outside the school and they want to know if it is true. They say that if I tell them it isn't, all will be forgotten and things will go on as before. I don't know what to do. Do they want me to lie? Nothing about all these years allows me to lie. I think I'm going to be sick.

I am expelled for two weeks. Stripped of head boarder, prefect, leader. I have to hand in my white blazer.

My Dearest Cath,

I know what you're going through. Though you brought this on yourself, you are being persecuted unfairly. Try to hold on to the power within you, it will carry you above all negative and hurtful troubles—this is the <u>Inner Secret</u>. Try to be <u>Positive, Loving</u> and <u>Kind</u>, as you always have been, for "<u>This too shall Pass</u>."

Ever your loving Dad

A fter high school I want to be a famous actress.

May 1, 1970

Dear Candidate:

Congratulations! You have been accepted into the two-year Theatre Arts Program commencing September.

I live at home for one year with my parents. Except for summers and school holidays I've never lived with them and it's a tight squeeze, but with classes and going out to plays, movies, and parties, I'm hardly ever home.

My classmates are artists—uninhibited, imaginative, creative, self-centered. They happily play a full range of emotions and characters both on and off the stage, comfortable performing in voice, dance, and role-playing classes. I want to be, too, but I'm not. They aren't bored with the classes on set, lighting, and costume design, prop construction, and stage management, but I am. There's a lot of partying going

114

on and everyone's having sex and I want to have sex too but I don't know what to do or say to boys.

I quit after a year. Soon after, I visit my mother, who is volunteering once a week in a busy downtown hospital, and watch the nurses in crisp white uniforms rush about, confident and certain. I want to be a nurse.

April 5, 1972

> *We are pleased to advise you that you have been accepted into the three-year in-hospital RN training program. Please see the attached sheet regarding uniforms. You are required to live in the hospital residence for the first six months.*

We eat in the hospital cafeteria and obey a nightly curfew. After six months we start to work full-time on the wards, wearing real nurse uniforms—starched white dresses belted at the waist and buttoned down the front, white nylons, white duty shoes, white caps. We rotate through all the clinical areas and on my way to the wards in the dark early mornings I pray I won't get the patients with the draining wounds or colostomies or the ones with metal rods sticking out of their bones. I spend a lot of time in the utility room hiding, gagging, always afraid something will go wrong, that I'll give the wrong drug or the right drug but the wrong dose or do something I shouldn't, forget to do something I should.

I visit my parents on my days off. They have a new building manager and during one visit he yells at me for using my key to get into the building.

"You shouldn't still have a key if you don't live here anymore. This isn't your home!"

I go upstairs, sobbing. My father gets up from the couch to see what's wrong. I'm embarrassed, he's never seen me cry. When he hears what's happened he heads downstairs. I follow.

"This is my daughter's home and she will continue to use her key for as long as we live here." My father speaks very slowly, punctuating each word as he taps his finger on the man's chest. "Don't—you—ever—talk—to—my—daughter—like—that—again."

My father, awarded the Military Medal and the Order of St. George while serving with the Canadian Royal Engineers in the First World War, goes to battle. For me. Next time I visit there's a new manager.

My dad and I have been having occasional lunches at his men's business club. He likes to hear about the wards I work on.

"I like geriatrics the best, and cardiology. Old people say the neatest things, but they just spend all day in their wheelchairs in front of the TV and some never get any visitors."

"Oh gosh, that's not right. We're all going to be old one day. They should be looked after the way we would want to be looked after, don't you think so?"

Late at night I study the heart's rhythmic beats, the four small chambers with their miniature one-way doors that let blood flow in and out, in and out. I try to decipher the electrical signals, the patterns, waves, timing, as the stylus scratches back and forth across the shiny white paper, like bird claws.

My mother's confusion escalates. She calls all night long convinced that she has to move out of her apartment and has no money in the bank, that people are trying to break into her condo. Frantic about all the things she can't remember. I don't know how to help her. We try drugs that make her dizzy, drugs that make her fall, drugs that don't make her better.

She is still upset when I go over in the morning.

"I'm trying to get hold of the manager to tell him I'm under threat of death. Do you know where that man is, you know the one, he looks like . . . ?"

"Um, the good man or the bad man?"

"The good man."

"He's still at the office."

"Oh. Where's the bad man?"

"He's dead."

For months she asks after her brother, her mother, her father.

"Where's Mother?"

The first time I think I should tell the truth.

"Gran's in Heaven, Mum. Remember?"

She looks up at me, whimpering.

"Oh no, not Mother?"

The next time a lie.

"She's away for a week with Grampy but they're coming home tomorrow."

"Well, I never. I'd like to have gone . . ."

Then a half-truth.

"I don't know where she is, but I'll find out."

She makes a face, doesn't believe me.

"Oh, Mum, I don't know where they are. . . . I just don't know."

"Don't cry, darling, don't cry. I was the only one who liked to garden with Dad and I was, of course, his pet."

"Really? How did you know?"

"I was always around his neck. Do you know where Mum is?"

"Shopping."

"She'll be so pleased to see the birds, won't she? When will she be here I wonder?"

"Tomorrow. She'll be here tomorrow."

"Oh how wonderful. By the way, do you know if Dad was pleased?"

"He was thrilled. He said he was so proud of you."

"Oh my . . ."

A Steller's jay lands on her balcony railing. Cocks its head right, left, right.

"I can stay here? This is my home?"

"Yes, forever."

"Will I get the birds?"

"Yes, all of them."

"I can't see how I would move from a place like this that I own and that I've been in for the last ten years and know it perfectly."

"That's right."

"And it knows me."

I dream I'm going to a party with all my friends. We're walking up a long cobblestone path, shadowed from the hot summer sun by whitewashed houses. One by one my friends go through a door into the party. I'm last in line and when I get there the handle is missing. I can hear music and laughing inside, and pound on the door. No one comes.

An old friend calls.

"How are things going, Cath?"

"I can't do this anymore."

"Yes, you can. You have to."

"I need to lie down with a man but not a lover."

"I'm opening the Zinfandel."

I go over, suddenly shy. He stretches out on the couch, pats the space beside him.

"Here, come on."

I lie next to him, my head against his chest.

"I couldn't do what you're doing, not for all these years."

"Neither could I."

"What are you eating these days?"

"Tandoori salmon pieces, chocolate, wine, sleeping pills."

S everal times a week, sometimes more, my mother and I go to the mall for lunch and sit in our favorite server's section, waiting for hugs.

"Hello there, Mrs. B. You look so beautiful today, sweetie."

The restaurant is full of gray hair, walkers, wheelchairs. My mother's having trouble remembering how to use utensils, how to get food from her plate into her mouth, turns her head away quickly when I offer her a French fry and jerks her head back as I tip the coffee cup to help her drink.

"I wish you would stop shoving that!"

My tears drip onto the ugly maroon tablecloth.

"Never mind, love, never mind."

I feel terrible for shoving the coffee, for letting her see me cry.

A middle-aged woman sits across from us. Her mother can't talk but they spend the whole lunch hour laughing as the daughter ties the plastic bib around her mother's neck, spoon-feeds her, wipes her chin. The daughter smiles and smiles. I hate her. After a while the daughter and mother don't come back. I imagine the mother, dead. Relieved they won't be back. Jealous.

I order my mother fish and chips and a cream-filled pastry, food my health-conscious mother never would have eaten.

"We were very unkind to someone in here, love. I mean, poetically. But I think they should get some new words for their vision."

She slides her tongue around the edges of the pastry, scooping out the cream. A gray-haired couple stops by to say hello. My mother beams.

"We could split another treat, couldn't we, love?"

"Okay. Which do you like better, the day or the night?"

"The night."

"Because?"

"I can hide."

"Lightness or darkness?"

"Darkness."

"Because?"

"I don't show up."

"Which do you like better, vanilla or chocolate?"

"Chocolate."

"Because?"

"It's a freer-upper."

"How do you feel you are doing these days?"

"I have low points that I can't help, they just snap and growl. Jack the fairy tells me to get up and get going. We're struggling all the time against human combative forces but I feel better, love. Always sort of . . . this. Just trying to steer out of it."

"You aren't unhappy?"

"No."

"Because?"

"I'm with you."

After lunch we window-shop up and down the mall passing other women pushing wheelchairs, mostly young girls from other countries. I smile and nod. Sometimes we pass middle-aged daughters like me. I look away. The mall is cold. I tuck a scarf around her neck.

"I jumped up like a startled gazelle and then the prayer comes around. You're the best daughter a mother could ever have."

"No, Mum. I'm . . ."

"Yes you are, yes you are."

I don't want to be the best daughter a mother could ever have. I want to wrap my legs around a man and rock through the night rather than all this mothering of my mother.

During nurse's training my real father's second wife tracks me down.

"He has cancer. He wants to see you—please come."

I haven't seen him for fifteen years. I don't want to go.

He's lying in bed dying from the lung cancer that's spread to his bones. I recognize him, even though he looks like a skeleton. I give him the two tins of turtle soup my mother has sent along.

"It was his favorite soup. There's no point in holding a grudge after all this time, is there?"

I sit and hold his hand. His fingers are long and thin, fleshless. His face pinched.

"Are you in a lot of pain?"

I plump up pillows, straighten bedclothes.

"It's not so bad. I shouldn't have smoked, I guess. I just couldn't help it. I tried to visit you at school but they wouldn't let me see you."

His wife makes tea.

"How is your mother?"

"Fine. She has her own boat, she loves to fish."

"Yes, of course. And your brother . . ."

I want to ask him what happened, what went wrong. Why he didn't want us or come to see us or send Mum money. Why he was mean to Hughie. I don't.

He's in so much pain and I'm afraid of his answers. Don't want any more versions. He dies the following week and for months I play out how our conversation might have gone.

"Please forgive me, I'm so sorry. I never meant to hurt anyone. I loved you all so much."

He always says the right thing.

In the cautious warmth of an April afternoon we sit out on my mother's balcony and listen to the happy hollering of children.

"Oh, the little darlings."

"Were you a good mother?"

"I think I was. I tried to be, lovey. I was not terribly brown or round or quick."

"What made you a good mother?"

"I adore babies."

"What do you adore about babies?"

"I like their unspoiled natures and their God-given ways."

"What happens when a child dies?"

"You have to find some coupons and then they'd be thrilled with you and look after you and dress you. I think Cath makes them work out of it in little leatherette shoes."

"Really? Have you ever been married, Mum?"

"Once too many times."

"Do you have any children?"

"No."

She looks at her watch.

"Hurry, Mother and Dad will be here soon."

"Oh, um, they called this morning and they can't make it today, because they . . . they all have colds."

"Someone might have told me."

"You were asleep and they made me promise not to wake you."

"What nonsense, I don't mind being woken."

"They'll be here tomorrow. Will you help me fold these table napkins so we'll be all ready for their visit?"

She asks after my grandmother over and over.

"Is Mother coming today?"

"Um, I think she's coming tomorrow."

"Oh . . . I wish she was coming today."

"So do I."

She purses her lips, frowns.

"Oh dear, are you having a little pout?"

"A little pout, maybe."

"She has a cold and thought she'd better come tomorrow instead. She doesn't want to give you her cold, Mum."

"I never catch colds, Hugh."

"Hugh? Do you know who I am, Mum?"

"Do you?"

I take my phone with me wherever I go, leave contact numbers with the caregivers, check voice mail, call every few hours. Friends tell me to turn off my phone, take a vacation, that my mother could go on for years and that I should live my own life. This is my life.

After my mother has been sick for a few years an old friend calls.

"I must visit. We all have so many happy memories."

He never comes. Family and friends begin to write my mother off, write off her changing mind.

"I just don't know what to do or what to say to her anymore. I'm sorry but it's really as if she died a long time ago, isn't it? I mean she's ten percent of who she was—"

"No! She's becoming more and more. She's one hundred percent of who she is."

Their visits, infrequent. Uncomfortable—for me. My mother is thrilled to see them.

"Hello, hello. How lovely! Did you see the birds? There were three people that got on that bus and they were Irish . . . no they weren't—two Irish, one English, and I don't know what they said or where they were going. All over hell's half-acre!"

They interrupt. Correct. Cut her off. Fill in words. Change subjects.

"Oh Jo, it's starting to rain. We should go."

"I wonder if Hugh . . . I want to see Uncle Hugh's new coat."

"Uncle Hugh? But he's—"

Shut up shut up shut up.

"Thank you for coming."

I close the door.

"Uncle Hugh's got a new, a new car. He got a four-seater. He got that yesterday."

"Are we related, Mum?"

"Not by blood. We're sisters, brother and sister."

"Do you feel well looked after?"

"No, not now."

"Why is that?"

"There's nobody here. Nobody nobody all the time."

I bring out a brownie thick with chocolate icing.

"There's nobody around all the time. I'm not used to talking to anybody anymore but I will one day.

I think I'll get better when I get up in the morning although I don't feel like it. I get a little bit dejected about the whole thing but if I woke up and got up I'd feel wonderful, if I felt wonderful. Love, where are all the others?"

"They're coming back tomorrow and they're bringing you presents."

"Really? They never forget do they, love?"

After graduating with my RN I work in hospitals for two more years and take night-school courses to get into university. I don't want to stay in hospital nursing, which I like but not very much. I'm queasy and worry about my patients all the time. I want to be . . . something else.

I meet a man on crutches at the Laundromat. He's got a handlebar moustache, is sweet, and likes me. We marry. I know we shouldn't and think he knows this too and that one of us should say so but we don't. I need a husband, need to be the sort of girl a man would marry. I don't know what he needs.

My husband and I spend a lot of time talking about our families.

"I don't understand why you had to go to boarding school when you lived so close to home."

"My dad had to travel a lot, I guess."

"Still, it wasn't fair."

One evening when we're over for dinner at my parents', I ask if we could please sit at the dining room table for dinner. My father heads for the den.

"I'm going to watch the news."

"Can't we just sit together for once like a real family and talk and not watch the goddamn news—you're such a big poop!"

My father turns and slaps me on the face, then pretends he's fooling around, sparring. Keeps slapping. I run down the hall to the bathroom. He comes down and knocks on the door—please will I let him in. He says he's so sorry, holds me tight. Starts to cry.

When we go back upstairs I can see my mother has been crying and my husband wants to go home but I talk him into staying. We go out for dinner.

Soon after we marry, my husband has surgery on a broken leg that won't heal. X-rays, physiotherapy, visits to the doctor, week after week month after month. He's in pain all the time. They need to rebreak his leg and bone graft the unhealing parts. I feel sick when he tells me what they're going to do. I hate the thought of messing about on bones with drills and hammers. Some of my nursing friends don't understand why I'm so upset.

"It'll be easy for you."

My husband and I make it for a few years. I pretend it's normal to live with someone, get up together in the morning, go to work, shop for groceries, come home, make a meal, do dishes. Pretend it's normal to spend evenings at home—reading, watching TV, talking about the day. We know we're not going to make it. I don't know how to get the man thing right and he drinks too much. I think he will stop drinking, that he will stop for me, and that my love will be enough. He doesn't. It isn't.

———

I finish my nursing degree and work as a medical research assistant. My husband knows how badly I want to go on to graduate school and he tells me to apply to all the best schools.

April 16, 1980

> *I am pleased to inform you that your application to the Johns Hopkins School of Hygiene and Public Health has been approved for admission to the Master of Public Health Program for the 1980–81 academic year.*

I move to Baltimore for a year and live in the International Residence, studying hard late into the night, seven days a week. My marks are high. I'm finally working my way out of the stupid class.

One Sunday I go to the free classical music concert held in the university auditorium. A Beethoven program begins with the Sonata for Piano and Cello in F Major, op. 5, no. 1.

I watch the pianist's face as she waits for the cellist's lead. Watch, as the lead switches back and forth between them, back and forth, like relay runners.

He leads, she follows, she leads, he follows. They tilt their heads toward each other, watching and listening . . . like a bird, head cocked, watches and listens for worms.

When I return home my husband and I don't talk, the bed is suddenly too small. We move away from each other quickly, our marriage over. A friend recommends work with the government up in the Arctic. A month later I find myself in the frozen North recruiting physicians to remote communities and trying to find ways to make them stay.

My father calls me every week and I tell him about my job, the northern communities I travel to, and the boards and committees I sit on. He offers suggestions on how to write and deliver a good speech and chair a meeting, how to manage difficult work situations—things my father knows about. He also writes.

January 20, 1982

Hi Cath:

The ability to think and speak on your feet carries through every facet of business. Stay with it, my dear. Many a time I've lectured myself in the mirror on the <u>Power of Positive</u>

Thinking. Remember to suggest what you really want a person to do—

Wrong: You wouldn't have Joe's phone number would you?

Right: You could let me have Joe's phone number couldn't you?

Your decision to go on to law school in a year or two is a good one and I agree that you'll be able to apply what you learn to any work you do. (I can't see you in a law office!) I know you want to fund this yourself but if you need $ I will help.

He has a clear head. I like this about my father.

I look up Vital Statistics—Death Registration and Certificates:

Event (Date): 1963 8 8 (Yr/Mo/Day)
Age: 13
Gender: male

Event.

I don't attend reunions at my second boarding school, but long after I've graduated I write to my headmistress.

"All those beautiful words, you saved my life. Thank you."

She writes back.

My Dear,

One day, when you are old, you will know how much your words mean. I am enclosing a quote that I think you will like, but cannot find the author's name:

"Surely the universe has by now shown us enough previously unsuspected wonders to occasionally accept, on faith, something we cannot yet explain."

Her beloved lifelong friend who also taught at the school is ill and no longer knows her.

It is terribly sad to see someone you love fail so rapidly. There seems so little I can do except try to keep her happy in her little home, and I feel I am not always successful in doing that.

We write back and forth over the months and she invites me to visit when next I'm in town—

So that we can both think again on the poems we once knew, and loved.

My headmistress dies before I do that. Sitting in her armchair in her own little home all dressed up for the wedding of one of her students, the speech she has been asked to give still resting in her lap.

I like to think of her in that chair, eyes closed, smiling.

During one of my visits home from the North my mother and I are browsing through family albums when we come across her wedding pictures.

"Do you remember that beautiful robin's-egg-blue dress you wore, Cath?"

"Oh, I loved that dress. And you in your ivory silk suit with the turban hat."

We move on to the album of my high school years—the grass hockey championship, boarders' birthday parties with huge flat cakes, my white prefect's blazer.

"Mum, I just don't understand why I had to go to boarding school. I mean, you and Dad lived right here in the city."

She freezes.

"Oh Cath, why are you still thinking about that? It was so long ago."

"Because I want to know. I was so unhappy there and you were unhappy about it too, Mum, I know you were. I just want to understand why I had to board. It didn't make sense."

She starts to cry.

"Dad was so much older than I was and he'd already raised a family. He couldn't work with children around the house, he needed quiet. He said he'd look after us and I thought it would all work out. I didn't know what to do."

"But he could have—"

"I hated that you were at that school but I didn't know what else to do."

"But Mum, you—"

"It would have meant the end of the marriage."

After three frozen winters in the North and three summers of endless light with evenings that never make it past twilight, I move to the prairies where the endless space of blue sky and golden earth stitch together tight against the horizon, and the warm sun-filled sky soaks through my skin, settling deep into bone and gut.

Law school. Constitutional Law. Legal Research and Writing. Personal Injuries and Compensation. Property. Contracts. Jurisprudence.

Law school classes are note-taking classes. We learn to be adversarial. I'd rather sweet-talk and I want to quit. My mother and I talk every few days.

"Keep going, love. But I must say it does sound dreadful."

Evidence, Criminal Law—everything reminds me of the killing of my brother. I learn there are different kinds of killing, that my brother was killed but not murdered, not as bad as murdered. Not as punishable.

Everything reminds me of the years I've spent hoping that the boy who killed him suffered, that he received the same sorrow-laden life sentence my mother and I did. I pretend he writes me a letter and says he's sorry. Pretend sorry will make everything better.

My dance teacher gives me a pep talk before competitions.

"Competitions are about having fun, not winning. It doesn't matter where you place, just have fun!"

I don't want to have fun. I want to be turned belly up and cut from vent to neck. Split wide open.

I buy a secondhand midnight-blue ball gown glittering with hundreds of zircon crystal rhinestones. Every time I wear the dress I pick up the scent of the other dancer's perfume. Pretend I'm her. Fox-trot, slow waltz, Viennese waltz—flying-around-the-room dances, wave-surfing dances. Layers of sapphire chiffon float up and down, up and down as we spin, spiral, and glide. The judges always say something nice and something constructive.

"Olé! Very dramatic. Tone your center for stronger balance on turns, and watch footwork. You display such drama. You were meant to perform!"

Most of the other competitors are better than I am and I'm not good enough to place at the top, but

I want to make it into the semifinals so I can dance all over again.

My mother loves watching the videos.

"Oh how lovely, a dress full of stars. Watch the timing, darling, you're a little fast on your turns."

My mother's face lights up every time babies come on the TV. I buy her a small comfy doll. She's the weight of a newborn, this smiling, happy baby.

"Yesterday I had her up on my lap around dinnertime and said a lot of soft words and nice things to her. I'm not very keen on being handed a lot of nasturtiums or something, you know. Especially black ones."

"I don't blame you."

"Did you hear about the chair in the fridge?"

"No, what happened?"

"When I went to take it out it fell apart in my hands. But to make things worse it was the other one, the other one, and she started making rituals to her in the other person's arms which happened to be raindrops, and started to criticize her so there was rain."

"Oh dear. How is your baby doll today?"

"I think we are quiet and sedated."

"She's lovely, you know."

"Because she's so beautiful. She's sweet."

"She looks like you. She has the same color hair."

"Boy, I'd like to look like that! But she's awfully tiny. I wish he'd sometimes get in the habit of giving her a hunk of beef or something like that."

"Oh, I gave her a hunk only an hour ago."

"Did she eat it?"

"Everything, every tiny bit."

"Then she must be pretty hungry."

"No, um, I think that's normal. I asked the doctor about it and she said the baby's weight is perfect. She's growing well and her weight is perfect."

"And did she mention anything about her weight?"

"Yes, she said her weight is absolutely perfect."

"Oh good. I don't think I can do it because she's not going to be alive. I'm thinking I'd love to have her. A little girl to run around, and you know, it would be fun I think."

A pile of crossword puzzles sits neatly stacked on my mother's bedside table. She's done crosswords all her life.

"I can't understand why they've changed these puzzles, love. They don't make sense."

I buy easy and beginner puzzles and glue covers from the hard puzzles onto the front of them.

"These are better now. There must have been some glitch."

After a few months she can't do any crossword puzzles.

My mother wants to know where I live.

"So you haven't been there for a long time, have you, dear?"

"Quite a while."

"How long?"

"I've lost track but quite a while."

"Have you? You never told us."

"I've always told you!"

"I never knew."

"Really? Where did you think I was?"

"I? Where did you think I was? Where do you think I—I don't know. God knows but he won't squeal because you came down here seventy-seven times in a row and stayed within a block of us and never let us know."

"Oh dear . . . I'm sorry, Mum."

"Never mind, love. Never mind . . . I don't know where my house is. Oh, I hate myself, I hate myself! I'm just talking nonsense. People keep moving things so I can't find them. I couldn't bear it if my mind went, I just couldn't bear it. I think I'm going crazy!"

"It's about time."

"What?"

"I love crazy."

"Really?"

"You can't get crazy enough for me."

"It would be nice if someone told the old people what's going on. This business has been on and off, on and off, and I feel rather soured by everyone and everything and am not amused by a kettle of fish."

"What do you need to know?"

"Are you sure I'm eighty-six?"

"Yes, how old did you think you were?"

"I didn't know whether I was going that way or that way."

"What did you think you were doing?"

"I thought I was going in-between, somehow."

A scientist friend and I discuss the God neither of us believes in.

"I can't very well be a scientist and believe in God."

"Tell that to Einstein!"

I tell him I still talk to God because He's good company not because I believe in Him anymore. We laugh.

We meet three years into my mother's illness when friends introduce us at one of his lectures. We get together every month or so for two-hour lunches. He tells me he has been sick but hopes to live long enough to finish his projects.

We talk about music, books, sailing (his), and dancing (mine). He describes the sequence of genes and I try to understand mutagenesis, protein structures, and rogue cells but never do. I explain school figures in dance and he tries to understand sway and contrary body movement but never does. I tell him my dancer-sailor friend thinks the slow fox-trot is the closest thing to sailing he's ever found. My scientist friend gets that.

Dear T:

Another great lunch.
1. *"Imagination is more important than knowledge." (Einstein)*
2. *"A mind too active is no mind at all." (Roethke)*
3. *". . . I want real things—live people to take hold of—to see—and talk to—Music that makes holes in the sky." (Georgia O'Keefe).*
   See you Wednesday!
   —CB

Dear CB,

1. *Einstein would not have been able to exercise his mind and develop his Theory of Relativity without enough knowledge of Newtonian mechanics to know that they did not explain everything.*
2. *As for Roethke, I don't know where he's coming from.*
3. *Georgia should have stayed with painting.*

He always walks me to my car and sometimes we sit together in the underground parking, listening to classical pieces we've been discussing—Delibes's

Lakmé, Bizet's duet from *Les pêcheurs de perles*, and Sibelius's Symphony no. 4.

We kiss, but that's all.

> *Dear Sweet Lady,*
>
> *I have been meaning to tell you, for some time, how much I admire you caring for your mother. I know, with your background, spirit, and energy, that there are many places it would be easier, less isolating, and more fun for you to be.*
>
> *In admiration, T.*

I wish our lunches would never end but they do. One day my scientist dies. No more emails, witty repartee, white wine, compliments. No more kisses in the car.

Midnight. My phone is ringing.

"Hello, Mum."

"This room—it's too small, too small."

I've told the caregivers that my mother is allowed to call me whenever she wants to.

"Oh hello, darling. Hello, hello. How you have several times said that. You should see her face when she's half-empty."

"Um, what? What, Mum?"

"What a horse's ass you are!"

"Should we sleep a little more and then go out for lunch?"

"Oh no, you're all mixed up. We're all going out, dear. We have plans and I'm afraid if you drop by you'll find us gone."

"But I . . ."

"Don't cry, lovey darling, don't cry. Sleep, sleep, sleep. 'Sleep knits up the ravell'd sleeve of care, the death of each day's life, sore labour's bath, balm of hurt minds.'"

"Your Shakespeare is wonderful."

"Thanks very much. Are we going for lunch now, shall I get ready?"

"It's still early, let's go back to sleep and I'll call when it's time to get up."

"But when will you call? What time will you be here? Shall I go downstairs now?"

She's forgotten about the wheelchair, that she can't walk.

"No, I'll call first thing, and I'll come up and get you."

"But I don't know where I'll be tomorrow. You might not be able to find me, I may be back at the other place."

"I always know exactly where you are."

"But how, love?"

"I have a file that tells me where you are. It's up-dated every two hours."

"That settles the question."

"I'll sing a little song to help you get back to sleep but you have to promise not to laugh if I'm off-key."

"I'll try not to."

> *"Jesus bids us shine with a clear, pure light,*
> *Like a little candle, burning in the night*
> *In this world of darkness, so we must shine*
> *You in your small corner, and I in mine."*

"Lovely."

"Thank you. Would you sing me a song or would you like me to suggest one?"

"No thank you, they've all been suggested."

"Do you still talk to Jesus, to God?"

"Sometimes. But you know, He never answers me. Tomorrow is going to be a red-letter day!"

"Really, why?"

"I'm going home. I'm going home."

When I'm not with my mother, I stay in bed for long solitary hours dreaming of the past.

My mind turns to snow and ice and the frozen stark North where nothing blocks the view. My wind-borne tears form miniature icicles, like stalactites. I let my eyelashes freeze together and pretend I live in an ice castle. Wet Arctic air inhales exhaust from chimneys, cars, lung-breath . . . exhales clouds of tiny ice crystals that hover in midair. I hike alone across frozen lakes at dusky noon in the middle of a minus-forty-degree Sunday and look out on nothing. As far as my eye can see, nothing. Everywhere.

The land is white-full.

Someone has draped white bedsheets mile after mile across the frozen lake. Houses, snowmobiles, landlocked boats form sooty punctuation marks against the blank canvas, suspending white.

There's no end point for my vision—I cannot stop the seeing. Unbearable, all this white beauty. I have to look away.

I move back to the coast after law school. Home by the sea, I dream of quilted rows of grain in green and gold and sun-scorched fields of dust.

I rent an apartment near my parents and work as a consultant, enrolling in evening classes in theater, mime, improv, and clowning. On weekends I entertain at children's birthday parties and street performances. Then my father gets sick and everything changes, turns direction. Stops.

He refuses to let anyone look after him other than my mother and me. Doesn't want strangers in the house, won't spend the money.

"He told me I could have anything I wanted, Cath."

"I guess he changed his mind."

After years of looking after him my mother is sick with exhaustion. We can't manage anymore and have to take him to a nursing home for veterans. We visit often. He's unhappy.

"I want to go home."

He sits on the edge of his narrow metal bed in green-striped flannel pajamas and a navy housecoat, eating

161

a chocolate chip cookie. He holds it with both hands, turning it clockwise, nibbling the edges.

"Good, good . . ."

"Dad?"

He doesn't look up.

"Dad? You shouldn't have sent me to boarding school. I wanted to go home every day for seven years."

"I'm confused."

"No, listen to me. I wanted to go home all the time too and I was just a girl. It wasn't fair."

We sit in silence.

"Dad? Dad?"

My father nibbles on his cookie, around and around.

My father is dying.

I wash his face, comb his hair, clean his mouth—and listen. All day all night long I listen to his sporadic, gurgling, labored breathing until at last there is no sound at all. I wonder if I will miss him. Stay missing how things might have been. Could never have been.

After my father dies my mother buys a condominium near her brother. It overlooks the water and the three of us often sit out on her deck and watch the sea.

"Oh boy, we'll be able to see boats from here all day."

"I'd like to rent a runabout one day, Jo. Put a line over just for fun."

"Oh, Hugh, let's!"

Then one day her brother's heart stops and when they start it again, his mind doesn't work properly. She spends a lot of time with him, mostly at her house so he can see the boats coming in and out of the harbor.

"Cath, pick up Uncle Hugh on your way over, dear, and we'll have an old-fashioned tea party."

She makes ginger creams and baked custard.

"Right out of Mother's old recipe book, Hugh. Wouldn't she be pleased?"

She wraps him up in a wool blanket, hands him the binoculars.

"Look at that big freighter coming in. I wonder where it's from."

He looks through the binoculars.

"Do you think the salmon are running, Cath?"

"I don't know, Mum."

My uncle has barely touched his food.

"Come on, Hugh, eat up."

"Stormy, Jo Jo. Not good."

"You're so thin, can't you eat another spoonful?"

"The sea's a rolling mess."

On the day her brother dies my mother calls to say she has sad news.

"But it's good. No more suffering for Uncle Hugh."

My mother and I sit side by side on her couch and watch the November wind whip leaves off the trees. We watch the sea as the days grow darker. Shorter.

"I wouldn't be alive if it wasn't for you."

"Don't remind me, Mum!"

"Aren't we amusing today?"

"Tell me about the sky."

"Oh, I don't know about the sky. It's pretty beautiful . . . but you have to wear gloves because it puts fingerprints on it and you don't want that."

The sea is pewter-punched. Moody. I straighten her blanket.

"Is your pillow comfortable?"

"Yes, it's six-eighths comfortable."

We listen to the radio.

"Is that Beethoven, Mum?"

"No."

"Could it be Chopin?"

"No."

"Because?"

"He's dead."

"Clever."

The announcer introduces Glenn Gould and *The Goldberg Variations.*

"Oh love, listen . . ."

"Do you like how he plays, Mum?"

"He was a genius."

I bring out her old piano music and open Bach's *Schafe können sicher weiden.* She places her hands lightly on the dining room table and mimes the melody.

"*La, la la la, la la la, la la la . . .*"

"Lovely. Oh my, here's 'Moon River.'"

She peers at the notes and I sing along with her playing.

> *Moon River, wider than a mile,*
> *I'm crossing you in style some day.*
> *Oh, dream maker, you heart breaker,*
> *Wherever you're going I'm going your way.*

I open a pack of chocolate-covered digestive cookies.

"What do you think of Bach?"

"I don't know if he was nutty but he was obviously odd."

"Mozart?"

"I think he should have his tonsils taken out and looked at."

"Beethoven?"

"Oh wonderful, but some parts of it were roaming off to different stages."

"Chopin?"

"Heaven can wait, this is paradise! La . . . la la, off to see the world, there's such a lot of world to see . . ."

"You have perfect pitch."

"I know."

"Which do you like better, the dark or the light?"

"Darkness."

"Because?"

"I don't show up. Darkness—and the light."

"Because?"

"Because I'm nervous."

"Nervous of?"

"Men."

"All men?"

"Amen! There were all these men around earlier."

"Really? Do you like having men around?"

"Yes."

"Because?"

"They look nice in their jockey shorts."

An accountant I know opens a clothing store because she doesn't want to work for other people anymore. Neither do I. I'm bored, and sick of wearing suits.

I open a baby store full of books, stars that glow in the dark, hand-painted baby gum boots, and furry creatures with shiny expectant eyes. For the next seven years I walk around my little shop, often with a newborn in a sling, telling stories to toddlers and soaking up magical little minds. My mother drives over two to three times a week to help me. We order lunch in, spend the day cooing and cuddling babies.

Every morning I'm greeted by the trees and birds and animals painted on the walls and ceiling. Before putting up the OPEN sign I play Loreena McKennitt's "Huron 'Beltane' Fire Dance." Turn up the volume. Dance a jig.

Are we related?"

"You're Elizabeth Oxenbury what will you do, what will you do. You are Alex-go-lightly, you are Miss Teryaki."

"What's my name?"

"Lorna Doone—no . . . well, your first name, second name or—?"

"The other name, the one you just called me."

"Harbinger."

"Harbinger of?"

"Harbinger of birds."

Every time I meet new people I have to explain about my brother.

"Do you have any brothers or sisters?"

"No."

"Spoilt rotten!"

Thirty years to settle on an answer.

"Do you have brothers or sisters?"

"I had a brother, but he died."

"How did he die?"

"He . . . I can't talk about it."

"I'm sorry. How old was he when he died?"

"Thirteen."

"Oh. That long ago?"

They always sound relieved. As if time meant something.

ove, I'm not going anywhere alone."

L "No, absolutely not."

"I think that's good, you only need to say, 'Mum, this is your own home, you'll always be here.' Something like that, it doesn't mean . . . and nothing is left vague. I think that sounds good."

"Okay. Mum, this is your own home, you'll always be here."

"When I look around at all these pictures I don't know how they did it, they must have taken all the pictures from home and had copies of them made and then put them where they were supposed to be put. I don't know, they must have made a lot of trouble. All the rooms are exactly the way that I am at home."

"That's right, Mum."

"I feel a lot better having spoken to you because before I really didn't know anything. I was going backward. Why or how or anything."

"Do you feel you have the right information now?"

"Yes, I think so. But I think I should go home now, love. It's getting late."

"Please Mum, this is your home . . ."

"You don't have a lot of spunk today, do you?"

"No. How did you know?"

"I just had a baby feeling. Don't go ruining your insides."

"How would I do that?"

"By being the eldest can of fool your mother has produced. At any rate it's going to be better now. You see, I'd rather be by you than anywhere."

"That's how it's going to stay."

"I slept well. No dark clouds."

"What happens when there are dark clouds?"

"My voice vanishes."

"Where does it vanish to?"

"Into my belly. Rumbles around."

"What happens when we die?"

"I don't know, I was never there."

"Will we see people we know?"

"I don't know and I don't know anyone who would."

"Where do we go when we die?"

"I'm going where I came from."

"How are you in general, do you think?"

"You mean, eventually?"

"Um, yes."

"Well, happy eight out of ten. You see it's my root section, and I can't let it down even if it lets me down. What happened to the joy of life, Cath?"

"I don't know, what do you think?"

"I think you thought it was going to be better than it was."

She eats a fudge brownie smothered in whipped cream.

"Boy, that's good."

"Your hair looks nice since you've had it cut for the summer."

"That wasn't my summer. Don't touch it, it might be microwaveable."

"I'm tired today. I think I'll head on home."

"And then are you coming back?"

"Well, I thought I'd stay home and then call you from there."

"Don't bother calling me to say you aren't coming back."

"Damn it, I come here every goddamn day! I just need to go home for a bit. I'll be back tomorrow, as usual."

My mother starts to cry.

"I'm such a nuisance, I wish I was dead."

"I wish I was dead too. And when I'm old there isn't going to be anyone left to take care of me."

"Oh love, don't."

"No one left who knows my story."

She cries and cries.

"I'm sorry, I'm sorry."

"I don't think I'm doing well, love. I think I'm a long-suffering person—can I help you with suffering? I'd like to. Maybe someone will turn the clock around."

"I'm just so tired, that's all."

"Poor Cath."

"Because?"

"Her mother."

I turn on the TV.

"I just wish someone would let the old people know what's going on."

We watch a woman decorating a bedroom in lime green.

"What an abortion. That woman transports ill-health."

On the way home I think about my brother.

"Goddamn it, Hughie—why did I have to be the one left behind?"

I sell my store and plan to take a year off to think about what's next.

I take my mother on a holiday in the sun. We stay in a desert resort surrounded by twelve-million-year-old boulder formations, gigantic cacti, and jackrabbits. The days are hot and dry, the nights, cold. We settle in for our first evening in front of a roaring fire.

"Love, this is the most beautiful place. I'm not nearly as achy here. I'm going to bed early, I want to be fresh for the tour tomorrow."

There isn't going to be a tour. On the second day of our holiday my mother gets sick and she gets sicker every day. We fly home. On the plane she closes her eyes, clenches her teeth. I hold her hand and watch her face, the sweat running down my back.

In the hospital she rushes back and forth to the toilet, the bright red blood swirls around and around. The doctor says my mother has a tumor in her gut. Sitting on her gurney I think about her dying, think I can manage and be strong as long as she doesn't suffer too much. As long as it doesn't go on too long.

It isn't a tumor, she isn't dying. She has small pouches in her gut that bulge outward like an inner tube poking through weak sections of a tire. They keep getting infected and she spends the next year with fevers and pain, on and off antibiotics, homebound, bathroom-bound. Sometimes she stays with me and is up and down all night long. I sit beside her as she rocks back and forth.

"What shall I do? Oh dear, dear. What am I going to do?"

She gets sicker and sicker. Everything changes, turns direction. Stops.

Christmas. She has major surgery and comes to live with me for a while. Late afternoons we watch the twinkling holiday lights on the balconies across the street and the headlights flickering back and forth on the bridge—the comings and goings of holiday parties.

During the day we scan the sea.

"Pass me the binoculars, love. I want to see what that tug is doing."

———

My mother decides to give up her driver's license.

"I hate this. I don't ever want to be a burden, love. Have I buggered your life? I'd hate to think I'd wrecked it. You'd have done all sorts of things if it hadn't been for me."

"I did all sorts of things before you got sick. I wouldn't change anything I'm doing now."

"Oh Lord, I would. You wouldn't have stopped the things you were doing just because of me, would you?"

"I wasn't doing anything when you got sick. I'd already changed direction."

"Then you were wrong."

Something has gone, something bad has gone. We've reached the limit of our soul of misery and we're now poof! We're just doing the best we can. We're not feeling like that, we just do, we just are. I think that's just the way it is."

"Our conversations are like excerpts from *Alice in Wonderland*, aren't they, Mum?"

"Yes. It's not as bad as it was, though."

"Oh no, it's nice. I love it."

"I think I'm more concentrated and, sort of. I sort of—am. It's become part of me."

"Shall we say good night soon?"

"*La la la—goodnight Irene, goodnight Irene, I'll see you in my dreams.*"

"You sure can sing."

"I felt free, Cath. I felt free and unhindered. I felt free as a bird. I like seagulls, they take off in a natural way—quite theatrical. Yes, free and undivided, like the sea."

"How are you like the sea?"

"I like to drown people. Certain people. No, but I feel refreshed, that I don't owe anyone anything.

———

Free to flap my arms like a bird and go where I want to go, do what I want to do. All I know is I've been zapped of my strength, yes, and all the funny little laughs. I've been zapped of them all. Zapped."

"Speaking of which, I'm pretty tired. I think I'll head home now."

"What? Why?"

"Why? I'm really tired, I have to sleep somewhere."

"Sleep? Have you got no bed up there anymore? I mean, have you got a bed up there? I can't even talk now. Have you got a bed up there? 'Not anymore!' says he. In other words I've destroyed the whole. I haven't got a bed up there. Are you down here to stay, love?"

"Well, I have a bed at home, is that where you mean? Where? Here? I'm not sure what you mean."

"It was quite plain, it was really quite plain what I asked you."

My mother likes to have her breakfast in bed now. One piece of whole-wheat toast with marmalade, and tea with milk from a two-handled plastic cup. She wears a pale yellow waterproof bib covered in purple and white violets and edged in rosy pink piping. When she sees me she laughs and claps her hands.

"Oh Hugh, I knew you'd come. I was praying you'd come. I've been waiting."

"Oh, I . . . yes, how are you, Jo?"

"I'll just get up and make us a cup of tea."

"Oh no, let me. How's my girl?"

"Fine, Hugh, as long as I'm with you. Oh yes, I always want to be where you are."

"You're my favorite girl, Jo."

"Oh boy, that's all I need to hear."

Some men like to talk when they dance. I nod and smile. Spew silent dysenteric streams of rage against the mirrored walls. Shut up! Shut up! I drag misery into the dance studio, stuck to the soles of my shoes. I don't want to talk when I dance. I don't want to listen. Shut up shut up shut up.

After the dance party I drive home. Most of the lights are out in my building. It's raining. The sweat on my back is cold and damp. I turn off the engine, sit back, grip the steering wheel. Start screaming.

My mother's in bed, propped up with pillows. I'm curled up beside her. It's a tight squeeze. Pillows to the north, under her head, pillows east and west under her shoulders and arms. South, under her knees. A lace collar circles the neckline of her now loose-fitting pink nylon nighty. She holds her baby doll against her right shoulder, nestled under her chin. From time to time she remembers it's there and nuzzles its forehead. Smiling, her eyes closed . . . the most beautiful gesture I have ever seen.

My mother's nose is running. I press a Kleenex up against her nostrils.

"Is that better, Mum?"

"Yes. Thank you, dear."

I leave two fresh pieces of Kleenex in her hand.

"Fly away, fly away, there you go, there you go . . ."

She has hold of the two pieces of white Kleenex and floats them through the air, up and down, up and down. They take on the perfect shape of wings. A white dove.

She watches the bird.

"There you go. Up, up, fly away, fly away . . ."

Prescriptions, creams, pills. Over-lit linoleum-floored drugstores. Bandages, potions. Liniment. I twist open the cap and dream of earth-scented, sweat-glistening flanks, the grainy warmth of horse breath inhaling, tickling, snorting, and a thousand pounds of horse drumming into the dusty earth in three-quarter time. No space between girl and horse, no room for sorrow, no spare breath for tears.

Now listen, lovey. I think if there was a tune or the right song, I could just go. Time is running out, that awful feeling of time running out is now backed up."

"Where would you go?"

"To Heaven, if God asked."

"That sounds wonderful. You could go fishing with Uncle Hugh. All the family would be there."

"There were mink up there you know, Cath. They tried to steal my bait! It was something else—the boat, the garden, and you and Dad."

"It sure was. Your garden and Dad's garden."

"His garden and my boat! Apart from my brother, um, my uncle, I can fish as well as any man. I could catch them so the men didn't like me. But I could, you know. Well, do you think that I should go? Do you want me to go?"

I want to say yes.

"I want you to go when you are ready."

I sit in a small pale examining room and look out at the day. Early spring blossoms are reaching for the sun—lilac, forsythia, a pink magnolia. I'm in my surgeon's office for the last visit before he replaces my left hip. There are a few plastic bones lying on the desk. I look away.

My surgeon's in his forties, easy on the eyes.

"How are things?"

"I've been praying for ovarian cancer."

"You what?"

"So I'd be dead before you have to replace my hip. I figured it was a fast cancer so I'd be dead before my name got to the top of your waiting list."

"What?"

"I know, it should have been melanoma, right?"

"You're kidding."

"No. I'm scared."

"Of?"

"Hospitals. Everything. I hate the idea of having my bones cut, it makes me sick."

"I pretty well have to do that if I'm going to fix your hip."

"I hate it!"

I'm not exactly shouting at him, but I want to. I want to blame him. Blame somebody.

I like that he has a shaved head, hope it means he's less conservative than most surgeons. Hope it means I can keep talking.

"I hate hospitals and being at the mercy of, of everyone, and I . . . well, I don't want anyone to see me naked on the operating table."

He raises an eyebrow. We smile.

"And I'm worried about the pain, what if I can't stand it? What if I'm not brave enough?"

"It's my job to take care of the pain."

I can't believe anyone will take care of the pain.

"I don't want to be on crutches and I don't want a bunch of stupid people in my home. This just isn't me. And my mother, she's been sick for six years, and is so mixed up now she won't understand why I'm not there. I really don't think I can do this."

"What about brothers and sisters?"

"No, I mean—there's just me now. Listen, I'm fine now. I'll go."

He stays.

"You need a plan. You need to get your mother organized with backup help. I'll fix your hip so you can dance again."

"But . . ."

"Something else?"

"I just need to do something before the anesthetic. I don't know. Maybe have some music on or . . . just something. Do you mind?"

My surgeon smiles.

"Do anything you want, sounds interesting."

Maybe I won't need cancer after all.

Saved voice messages from my mother on my cell phone—twelve. Saved voice messages on my home phone—seventeen.

"Press nine if you want to save this message. Press seven if you want to delete it."

I press nine every ten days. Her voice—clear garbled breathless funny frantic. Messages I can't bear to listen to again. Cannot erase.

No turning back. Too much pain. Starting-the-day pain. Ending-the-day pain. All-night-long pain. Year after year teeth-grinding driving-me-crazy pain.

I get back in touch with God.

"Please God please I'll promise anything if you stop the pain I'll stop wishing my mother was dead I'll stop wishing I was dead please God please."

I don't tell her about the surgery. She thinks I'm going to a dance competition in London.

"When are you going to London, love?"

"In a few weeks, Mum."

I write out letters for the caregivers to read to my mother while I'm gone.

Dear Mum,

Here we are in jolly old England. The weather is wonderful and you should hear all the English accents! Tomorrow we go to Bath. Miss you, all is well.

Love, Cath

For days, we talk about my trip to England.

"I want to do something for you. To pay for something. I've been sitting here worrying about it."

"Some pounds would be great, thank you."

"How do I get pounds, Cath?"

She starts to cry. Why did I say pounds? Stupid, stupid.

"Don't worry—I'll just go to the bank for regular money."

"What bank? How do I get there? Who has my money? I know the one girl who does but what was the name of the other girl, you know the one, there is something red, to do with red, you know?"

"I can't remember her name, either."

"Are you going away, love?"

"Yes, to London, to a dance competition."

"Oh? Can you do that? You'll need some money."

Body pain, alone pain. I wish someone would hold me, rock me. Whisper, "There, there, Cath." Grandmother-words. Mother-words. No one's words.

My mother and I talk up and down, back and forth, around and around. Can't breathe with all this talking. I try to find words that will ease her worry and stop her tears but I can't.

"Is there anything else you want to talk to me about before I go?"

"If you're old and feel like hell, wouldn't there be a part of you that would want things to end? I don't think it's a natural want, if you've got a disease, that you have to get someone to initialize it and then get someone to chop it off, do you?"

"No. I don't. Is there anything more you want to tell me as a sort of summary before I go away?"

"In summary I don't think there's anything more we can say because everything we want to know is really on there, who is in charge and what they're doing and all the rest, so I think that's about it. It sort of ends the story right now, for now, don't you think?"

"Yes."

"Going all the way to London, you'll probably meet a man. Are you fifty-one? I thought you were sixty-one. God, I'm awful. I can't remember anything. You look about thirty-one, perhaps. You're my baby. *My baby don't care for clothes, my baby don't care for clothes, my baby just carries on, la la la dee dah.*"

"Is it possible to find a man who will be a good husband?"

"I think the answer is yes, if you look in the right places."

"How do you do that?"

"I don't know."

"What makes a good husband?"

"Love."

"What is love?"

"Affection of your children."

"Well, I probably won't meet a man this trip but sometimes I do get tired of being alone."

"Oh, I don't know. I think it's a shame, but when you are alone I think that you're happy. You'll have to accept the fact that sometimes you are alone and sometimes you are not and that when you're not alone it means there's somebody there who's talking and everything. And well, you have to pray for the good and the bad at the same time. You can't have everything perfect the way you want and you'll find, probably, that you like it better the way it is."

My mother sips her tea. Smiles.

"London! That is something for you, isn't it? Aren't you a lucky girl? Wait till Mother hears!"

Sometimes I pretend I'm the one lying by the side of the road in the dark with everyone around fussing. I never think about the part just before dying, the bad part. I think about when it's over, the blackness, the quiet. The nothing. The best part.

We're watching Oprah.

"She's got all her marbles."

"She sure does. Are you warm enough, Mum? It seems colder today, doesn't it?"

"We'll have to have a fire in here when they come and they'll have to have a little fire in there. You can't have no fire, they dance by the fire."

I turn on the electric fireplace.

"Mum, where is Heaven?"

"Today it looks all the way around but I know it isn't."

"You know, my cat is sick and I need your advice. I'm worried about looking after him when I'm away at the dance competition. What should I do? I don't know what to do."

She puts her cup down, sits up straight.

"Do you know what I would do? I would make up my mind that you're not going to put your little kitty cat through any more trouble. He's had lots and he's running around and he's been pretty good, hasn't he?

I don't think it's fair to keep him running on that all the time, do you?"

"No, you're right. But it's a big loss."

"I know it is, love. You don't want him given stuff that makes him sick and groggy and all the rest of it just to keep him alive. . . . They do it and I think that's cruel. It's a good way to lose him now, he didn't go just because he was in the way, he went because he was ill."

"Yes."

"He's got two puppies anyway, two dogs—a nice one that you've got to keep won't you, for the time being?"

"Yes. What do you think we should do if an animal, or someone we love, dies?"

"Wipe the tears off your face and get going. Some things die younger than others, love."

"Why is that?"

"Their father."

"What do you think happens to animals when they die?"

"They go back to their roots."

"What are their roots like?"

"They're quite bright."

"How do they find their way back?"

"In their organs. They sniff and smell their way back."

Men complain that women try to lead and that's why we go the wrong way on the dance floor, why feet get stepped on. I go the wrong way because I'm afraid of doing something stupid or because I miss the lead signals. I don't know how to do nothing. Be empty enough, quiet enough inside to wait. To listen.

I can't believe someone else will take care of the leading. Take care of anything.

July. Disinfectant and stale linoleum, the stinking smell of hospital. Outside the sun is warming up the day. Inside, I'm lying on a cold gurney wondering where to put all my fear. In the bed next to me is an older man and through a thin beige curtain we share the details of each other's problems and the surgeries that are going to make them go away. I need his help.

"How's your handwriting?"

"Pretty good."

"I need to write something on my back and I can't reach, will you help me?"

"Sure! Come on over."

I shuffle over in my hospital-green kneesocks, holding closed the back of my thin gown. I show him the words penned all over my body.

"Wow!" He reads each one out loud:

"Dance is the hidden language of the soul." Martha Graham, right arm.

"I'll tell you how the sun rose, a ribbon at a time." Emily Dickinson, right leg.

"I came to live out loud." Zola, left arm.

No writing on my left leg, my surgeon initials that one so the wrong hip doesn't get replaced.

"Can you write my favorite Rumi quote on my back—'Sell your cleverness. Buy bewilderment.'"

He likes that one best.

"My surgeon said I could do anything I wanted."

We hug.

It's so cold. Two nurses wheel me down the hall to the holding room and I think about cattle trucks and slaughterhouses—regret refusing a sedative. There are a lot of people in the operating room, gowned and masked. I can't see their faces. I don't like being the only one in a thin cotton gown with no underwear on. A nurse is busy with instruments, unwrapping, counting, sorting. She lays out screws, metal plates, drills, hammers, chisels, a saw.

When I wake the pain has gone.

On the orthopaedic ward the nurses are dressed in various uniform styles and colors. Most wear pale pastel pantsuits in yellow, green, pink, and blue— baby-sleeper colors. There are no regulation starched white cotton uniforms, white nylons, white duty shoes, crisp white caps, no head nurse in charge. The ward runs down the full length of a pasty green hall with rooms lined up on each side. I've asked for a private room so I can have a phone, so I can call my mother. They wheel me into a room for three.

"I have to have a phone because my mother is confused and thinks I'm in England running a dance competition. Please, please can you get me a phone?"

My nurse is busy, tired.

"I'd have to borrow a portable but I might not be able to get one—"

I start to cry. She brings the phone.

"Mum? It's Cath."

"Oh love, I've been waiting for your call all day. Where have you been?"

"In England, organizing the dance competition."

"Oh how lovely, darling. Is it wonderful?"

I can't think, want to sleep.

"Yes . . . wonderful."

"What will you be doing, love?"

"Oh, tomorrow we go, um, we're going to Stratford-on-Avon, where Gran was born. I might not be able to call from there."

"Oh you must call. You'll try, love, won't you?"

"I'll call, Mum."

"I want to cut some of the brambles down, some of the old stuff. I've got something I could talk about but it's not nice so I won't but it's interesting—I dreamt last night that I had come back here from being up in the valley of a thousand deaths."

Click-click, I press the morphine drip. No matter what happens there isn't anything I can do for my mother today.

Click-click.

On the third day, I move to a private room and entertain a constant parade of visitors. I hate visitors in my home but want friends in my hospital room all day and night, competent friends who know how things should be, like doctors and nurses. I'm afraid that something will go wrong, that someone will give the wrong drug or the right drug but the wrong dose or do something they shouldn't, forget to do something they should, that they might not do things well enough. I need advocates, witnesses. I know bad things can happen in hospitals. Things much worse than dying.

Mum Mama Mutter Mother Nonna.
I never ask how long this could go on. How long she could last. I hear seventy-year-olds still grieve the loss of their mothers and fathers and I'm afraid.

Moeder Mamacita Maman.

When I get home from the hospital I want to be alone but I can't manage on crutches, can't carry food, plates, a cup, and I'm afraid of falling in the shower. I call my mother. I wish she was here, she'd know what to do.

"Where are you, love?"

"Still in England."

"In England? What are you doing there?"

"Organizing the dance competition."

"Oh, how lovely! You sound like you have a cold, love. Cath, I know where you'll meet somebody."

"Where?"

"In London! By golly by George, you'll marry! I think an English accent, if it's mild and it's just natural, well, it's very attractive—'Oh hello, oh I say, don't you look lovely tonight. Oh, would you like a cup of tea?'"

"Good accent. Why do you think people marry?"

"For two reasons—they want to fill up their boots, and they want to keep on going and they don't care where."

"What is love?"

"The blending of two souls."

"And?"

"It is the sublime, felt between two people in the same working order. I'd like a man who is singular of purpose and proud his purpose is legitimate and then we'll back him up."

"How would you know if the love that you felt for a man was true, it was right, and not in error?"

"I would think that you would know. I don't think you'd be worrying about whether it was right or wrong, I think you would know that it was just a one-man dealing, wouldn't you?"

"What do you do if you love a man and he doesn't love you?"

"Try somewhere else. But you're going to meet the most marvelous man in London."

"I am?"

"Well, it's not too late, is it? But it's getting there."

I dream I'm alone in the cockpit of a cargo helicopter. Something bad has happened and the pilot's gone, the engine's quit. I try my own keys, frantic to find one that will start the engine. Finally my mail key works. I put on the headset and call for help.

"MAYDAY—MAYDAY—MAYDAY."

The mouthpiece is broken off. No one can hear me.

I'm still on crutches for the first visit to my mother's.

"What in the world are those for?"

"My hip was sore, but it's all fixed now."

"What? Did you think to tell me?"

"I'm sorry, but it's good now. Does it seem like I've been away a long time?"

"I have been away."

"You? Where have you been?"

"Waiting for you."

"What was that like?"

"Not so good, she didn't wait very well."

"Who is she?"

"The one just eight years old and couldn't wait anymore."

Sometimes my mother has trouble talking and I can't understand what she's saying. She speaks in a jumble of words, I answer in a jumble of *hmms* and *ahs*. Other times she has no trouble speaking at all.

She no longer remembers how to dial the phone. No longer makes her starting-the-day calls thirty-calls-a-day calls ending-the-day calls middle-of-the-night calls. I wait all night long to answer a phone that no longer rings.

Hello? Hello?

I'm trying to get my mother's attention, make her see me, coax her back into my world. She's playing hardball. I know I should leave her be.

"Mum? Mum?"

She picks at her apron, folding tiny, perfect accordion pleats over and over. I move to a chair directly in front of her so she'll have to see me. Her eyes avoid mine, dart all over the room. Beautiful sea-green eyes. I lay my head in her lap and rest her hand on my forehead.

Judge Judy is on TV tackling cases and solving everyone's problems. I wish she were here.

My mother strokes my forehead, pulling fine strands of my hair with gentle staccato tugs. Her fingers dance across my face like little fairies tap-tap-tapping on a windowpane.

I try for the English accent of her mother.

"Hello, love."

Nothing.

The voice of her brother.

"Hallo there, Jo."

This triggers a smile and she looks down at me.

"Hallo there, Hugh."

Looks away. She spots her baby doll sitting in the chair across the room.

"Ah, hello my little love. What a darling boy you are. Yes you are, yes you are."

I bring her the doll.

"There you go, love. There, there. Mum's little love, aren't you?"

She closes her eyes. Her face radiant.

Christmas. Most of my friends are out of town. My mother is dying.

<u>Day One</u>

Our doctor visits, gives advice, support. I tell her I didn't think Mum would be able to speak so well.

"Sometimes at the end people become very clear."

She writes prescriptions, listens to my mother's chest.

"Her heart is still strong. We have a way to go."

Birthing words.

For dinner I feed my mother pieces of milk chocolate, custard, sips of cold white wine.

"Mmm . . . good. Mum and Dad were over this morning and they just love my new place."

"Wonderful. Do you know who I am?"

"You're my baby. You're my step, step away."

The home-care nurse visits, inspects, arranges, and starts an IV for me to put drugs into. Listens to my mother's heart. I wish someone would listen to mine.

I lie beside my mother's struggled breathing, her wet, constant cough. Pat her chest.

"Is there enough compassion in there?"

"Yes, Mum. It's full, beautiful."

"Oh, good."

"Is your hand bothering you?"

"No, not really. Why?"

"You're rubbing your fingers."

"It's much better than last night. Last night, this finger here was giving all the answers."

Day Two

"Mum, are you looking at something? Is there someone in the room with us?"

"No."

"That's good."

"Just a little bird."

I straighten her bedclothes, give her a sip of water.

"Where's Mother?"

"She's coming first thing in the morning. She's been baking all day just for you but you mustn't let on, she wants it to be a surprise."

"I wish she were here now . . ."

"So do I."

———

I turn on the radio.

> *We wish you a Merry Christmas,*
> *We wish you a Merry Christmas,*
> *We wish you a Merry Christmas, and a Happy*
> *New Year.*
> *Good tidings we bring, to you and your kin . . .*

Turn it off. I look through her music and choose a Chopin prelude, op. 38. My mother closes her eyes, waving her hand left and right, in perfect time.

"Listen, there isn't any room for the melody . . ."

I take her hands and kiss them. Breathe them in. Fine, ladylike hands. Octave-reaching hands. Reeling-in hands.

"*La la la, La la la, La La, La La . . .*"

On her last trip to the bathroom she is frail, shaky. Her thin legs dangle high above the floor like a child's. The back of her hair lies flat against her head. My mother looks up, smiles.

"My great big love, aren't you?"

My mother is restless. All day long and through the night she talks to people I cannot see.

"Are there people in the room?"

"Yes."

"Do you know them?"

"I don't think so."

"Would you like me to ask them to leave?"

"Oh no, it's fine. They'll leave soon, thank you."

Every four hours I give my mother injections to ease her pain and restlessness. I put them into her IV, sometimes into her arm, trying to find a place that won't make her wince, but she always winces. I stroke her brow, give her ice chips to suck on, lift the thin damp strands of hair off her face. I've sent the caregiver away. I want to be alone with my mother.

"I'll tell you something. . . . Cathie and I are covered in flowers."

Day Three

Our doctor visits.

"It won't be today."

I start to cry.

"I don't think I can do this anymore, I can't bear it."

"Yes, you can. I know you can. You can call me whenever you want to. You're doing a great job, it won't go on forever."

But it does.

The flowers I've ordered arrive—three stems of deep pink, frilly-edged orchids and a dozen roses—bright red, tinged with orange.

I give my mother the drugs that are supposed to take away her moaning but they don't. I run my hand over her brow, back and forth, cooing, stroking, nodding.

"There, there now."

I wish someone competent were here, a take-charge sort of person, an English nanny. I wish someone would hold me. A man. My mother.

Day Four

My mother is struggling to breathe. I listen to her trying to catch her breath and have trouble catching mine. I make myself tea and take the steaming cup out onto the balcony. A sliver of December sun catches my face. A crow sits on a branch a few feet away.

"Pretty bird, pretty bird . . . you beautiful thing, you."

I go back inside and call my bravest friends to sob out the horror of my mother's dying.

"I don't know what to do. I can't stand it anymore."

They tell me it will end and that I'm doing all the right things but no one can tell me how to stop my mother's suffering, no one can tell me why my mother has to suffer.

Day Five
The doctor comes.

"Not long now."

My mother is a skeleton. Her face has angles I haven't seen before. By late afternoon there's a large red blister on her back. I call the home-care nurse, screaming.

"I was a nurse and I can't even take care of her!"

"No, no, it happens almost all the time, no matter what you do."

"I haven't turned her enough, haven't taken proper care of her skin. I haven't done anything right!"

"You've taken wonderful care of her and she can't feel anything now, it's all right."

It isn't.

I look out the window at the dark, empty street. My mother is breathing through her mouth and no matter what I do I can't keep her mouth and lips moist. Pieces of skin come away with each bloody lemon-flavored swab. She clamps down, won't let go. I start to cry.

"I'm sorry, Mum. Please, let go . . ."

Day Six
My mother is no longer awake. I watch her chest rise and fall in thin, uneven gasps and try to follow the

shallow rhythm, in-out in-out, but I can't get enough air. It's almost midnight.

Her finely shaped lips change from berry-stained to light rose to lavender, settle on a soft smoky gray, like the underbelly of a jellyfish. I kiss her forehead, her hollow cheeks.

"There, there, Mum. Almost over. It's good, soon no more suffering."

There are long seconds when my mother doesn't breathe. I hold my breath and listen—was that my mother's last breath, was that her last breath? Was that my mother's last breath?

And then—there is no sound.

I lay pink orchids and crimson roses on my mother's chest, cradled in her arms. In amongst the blossoms I slip two photographs, one of my mother and me, the other of Hughie, smiling. Lastly I tuck in a spool of twenty-five-pound-test fishing line.

Her baby doll is staying behind, with me.

The woman at the spa greases down my hair then rubs my skin with a rosemary-scented oil, binding me tight with Saran Wrap and a warm blanket.

"I'll be right outside, all right?"

"Yes, I'm fine."

After my mother dies a friend gives me a gift certificate.

"This will be so good for you."

I close my eyes and try to relax but I hate the rosemary, hate that I can't move my arms. I think about roast chicken, the hens on my uncle's farm. My mother, bound in white. I can't breathe and start to cry.

"Excuse me, hello?"

She rushes back in.

"I'm sorry, I didn't know I would panic. I never panic."

She brushes her hand across my forehead.

"It happens a lot."

"It's my mother, she—"

"Let's get you unwrapped."

My mother is gone . . . I want to say. She wipes a piece of hair off my cheek and places a cool cloth over my eyes.

"Thank you, Mum. I mean—"

We both laugh and she leaves the room, keeps the door ajar.

I whisper into the pungent darkness.

"Mum. Mum. Mum."

I'm having my nails done. I want to look nice for my mother's memorial. I call a friend.

"I'm picking up her ashes next week."

"Oh."

He changes the subject, talks about the weather, work, our friends. Nothing talk. I make a note to take him off my ash-telling list. My list of anything-telling.

My hands soak in the warm, soapy water and I can't stop crying.

"I'm sorry. . . . You see, my mother died. I'm having my nails done for her service. My mother is gone."

She looks at my quivering mouth. Looks away.

The last three and a half pounds of my mother sit on a shelf in my bedroom closet, tucked inside a gold satin jewelry box. I know I should do something with her ashes, scatter them out at sea . . . but I can't. I crawl into bed, lay them on my chest.

She's cut me loose. No more home-care stores, Seniors' Daycare Centre, wheelchair pushing, lifting, getting in and out of the car, frantic trips to the toilet, lunches at the mall. No more poetry.

"Any news, Mum?"

"Cathie was up here and she said to me, 'Mum, I'm not going to offer to give them my shadow.'"

"Where was this?"

"Somewhere . . . on the other side of here."

August, four in the morning. I water and fertilize my orchids—*Phalaenopsis, Dendrobium, Cymbidium*—then sit out on my balcony in the retreating dark and wait for cruise ships. Across the street four deserted shipyard buildings stand naked, their skeletal frames picked clean. Pieces of torn black plastic, like shredded bat wings, whip irritably in the wind.

A flock of gulls performs synchronized flight patterns against the growing light, banking left then right, around and around. For a split second as they turn there are no birds at all.

Three geese fly low over the slate-gray sea in perfect V formation as one by one the ships come into view—*Norwegian Sun, Zuiderdam, Seven Seas Mariner*. Hungry seagull chicks screech on the roof next door as the first ship slides silently across the glassy calm of the morning sea.

The weather channel on my marine radio predicts a trough of low pressure well offshore moving slowly toward the coast. Moderate southeasterlies increasing to strong. A chance of rain. An orange-hulled freighter forges through the choppy standing waves of the tide rip.

It's coming in too full, you can't see the Plimsoll line.

March. I'm early for my appointment. Bulky black photo albums full of artwork line the shelves. Dragons, hearts, butterflies, anchors. I listen to the heavy drone of rock music and a high-pitched buzzing coming from behind a white screen. Young people come and go.

My artist doesn't like the sketches.

"We can't use these."

I tell him I want to get started.

"Right now? No stencil?"

For weeks I've been sending him emails with stories about birds, rivers, dance.

"You understand what I want."

"Yes."

I wonder what the pain will be like, if I'll be brave enough. Except for the light shining on my back, the room is dark. The two of us, wordless.

The needle burns. I think about dance. Breathe in-2-3, out-2-3, in-2-3, out-2-3 . . . around and around. We take a break every thirty minutes but

I don't look in the mirror. After four hours I can't breathe in waltz time anymore and start clicking my heels together, rat-a-tat-tat-tat-tat-tat, rat-a-tat-tat-tat-tat-tat.

"Can you last fifteen more minutes?"

"I don't . . . yes, I think so."

I don't cry but I want to. Ten minutes later the buzzing stops. I sit up, dizzy. In the mirror—a bird. Carved on my back, a black-edged bird. Raven? Hawk? Unnameable.

I spend a lot of time looking in the mirror.

"There you go, there you go. Fly away."

Bird cocks his head, blinks. Stays.

Most of my friends are horrified.

"What if—oh my God it takes up half your back!"

"Are you crazy, it's going to be with you the rest of your life!"

Claw-tickling in the middle of the night. In the morning I look to see what he's written. Bird uses invisible ink.

I listen to my heart, lub-dubb, lub-dubb. Bird listens too, paces back and forth, left foot, right foot, left foot. Rocking, limping . . . dancing.

We spin, spiral, and glide . . . weightless into the night where there is nothing.

Everywhere.